Put On Your
Big-Girl Shoes

My dear Rena —
There are no words
to express my thanks to
you.
   It is my deep honor
and privilege to share
your story and to have
you as my new
Treasured friend!
Thank you for teaching us
all about compassion &
purpose in this life!
      with deep affection &
gratitude.   Lori xo

Put On Your
Big-Girl Shoes

Stepping into Courage, Resilience, and Gratitude

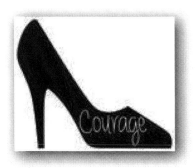

Lori Stevic-Rust Ph.D.

Integrated Press

Integrated Press
Copyright 2016 by Lori Stevic-Rust Ph.D.
All Rights Reserved. Published 2016
Printed in the United States of America

ISBN-10: 0998147206
ISBN-13: 9780998147208

Cover Design by Trevor Blosser
Cover Photography by Laura Watilo Blake
Editing by Katrin Schumann
Copyediting by Ursula DeYoung

Dedicated to women around the world who courageously step into their confident, big-girl shoes, push through fear, and find the strength to walk empathically in the shoes of each other, fighting injustice and living with purpose.

"You've always had the power my dear, you just had to learn it for yourself."

— GLENDA, *THE WIZARD OF OZ*

Praise for Put on Your Big-Girl Shoes

"This book is a powerful collection of stories about women finding courage and resilience in the face of adversity. Each story is a poignant reminder of the power women have to create positive change, including the story of NDI staff member Andi Parhamovich, who was a young and courageous advocate for democracy and women's political leadership. The Andi Parhamovich Fellowship, established in her name by NDI and the Andi Foundation, continues her legacy of dedication to women's empowerment worldwide."

-- Madeleine K. Albright, former Secretary of State and Chairman of the National Democratic Institute (NDI)

"I survived because one person saw what others refused to see. I hope that reading my story, as told in this beautifully written book, will give new life to each of you--so that you discover your own moral courage and ability to stand up for each other."

---Rena Ferber Finder, Holocaust Survivor from Schindler's List

"Every woman needs to know that the insecurity we sometimes feel is universal - we all have moments where we question our talents, capabilities, intelligence etc. But we also need to know how to overcome those moments. That's what we learn from Dr. Lori. I love these women she introduces us to because they help us understand how to tap into our authenticity and find the courage to examine ourselves, imperfections and all. I've learned that comparison is the thief of joy...but sharing our stories isn't about competition. It's about lifting each other up and recognizing we're already equipped to do whatever is necessary to make things right in our lives...we've just forgotten that truth. Dr. Lori and

these women will remind you that you're stronger than you think...and no matter what you've been through, there's a purpose for you.

--- Christi Paul, CNN New Day Weekend Anchor, HLN anchor/reporter & Author of "Love Isn't Supposed to Hurt"

"Written by clinical psychologist Dr. Lori Stevic-Rust, "Put on Your Big-Girl Shoes" is based on the lessons of highly successful women that were collected by the author over years of overcoming her own personal challenges. From these women's narratives, we learn about the importance of authenticity, finding balance, facing our fears, overcoming tragedy, healing, empathy, and finally, standing up for others. These women's journeys through self-discovery, courage and resilience teach us how to make a difference in the world and how to live a purposeful life. This book is the ultimate guidepost for bringing out your best self."

---Elaine R. Martin, MSLS, DA, Director, Francis A. Countway Library, Harvard Medical School

"Put On Your Big-Girl Shoes by Lori Stevic-Rust is a book you won't be able to put down. This hand-book for life is a testimony of truth wrapped in total transparency. *Put On Your Big-Girl Shoes* will rewire destructive tapes rolling around in your brain and set you on a corrective course that will take you to a higher level of influence, true authenticity, joy and power. You will be changed and you can thank Lori."

---Margaret Mitchell, President & CEO of YWCA Greater Cleveland

"Real women, real stories and real inspiration for those who are courageous enough to "put on their big-girl shoes." Dr. Lori Stevic-Rust takes you on an emotional, fascinating journey from fear and self-doubt to strength and resilience."

---Micki Byrnes, President & General Manager, WKYC-TV

"Dr. Stevic-Rust gives women real-life examples of what strength and courage really look like today, whatever a woman's life situation and challenges. In this era of pessimism, she spreads optimism. Watch out: this book might change your life."

---Katrin Schumann, Author of "Mothers Need Time Outs, Too" and "The Secret Power of Middle Children"

"How I would have appreciated Dr. Lori's book had it been available thirty years ago—I could have avoided being victim to the "Imposter Syndrome." Dr. Lori demonstrates the power of storytelling in her compelling book, "Put on Your Big-Girl Shoes," by allowing readers to experience the same feelings of self-doubt as she does, but then showing us example after example of how we can tap into our own resilient, authentic selves and grow up. I was particularly moved by the story of Rena Finder, one of the Jews saved by Oscar Schindler. Dr. Lori does a masterful job of illuminating three key themes of the book–finding gratitude, the power of empathy and becoming an eyewitness–in her sensitive recounting of their meeting. This is an important read for everyone, women, and men, too, who want to learn how to not only become more confident, effective, and successful in their own lives, but also how to truly make a difference in the lives of those others whom they ultimately serve."

---Hedy P. Milgrom, Senior Vice President and Chief Development Officer, Jewish Federation of Cleveland

Foreward

As I stepped on to the elevator—wearing a form-fitting dress and three inch heels—I felt a sense of calm, excitement and a tad nervousness all at once. It was 9:30 AM on Wednesday, September 8th, 2016 and I was at the Hilton Cleveland Downtown, about to be interviewed by Dr. Lori Stevic-Rust. I knew she was going to ask me to talk about my personal story of overcoming my childhood struggles with crippling shyness... about how I went from dreading having to speak up, to becoming a public speaker at ease with vast crowds.

Just the previous day, I'd delivered a standing-room only Facebook video marketing session at Content Marketing World, a widely popular event with over 3,000 attendees. This type of environment has been my comfort zone for the past fifteen years. And, speaking to businesspeople about Facebook is my wheelhouse – I love, and align with, CEO Mark Zuckerberg's mission: to make the world more open and connected.

Yet, I find that how people relate through Facebook can be strained: superficial at times yet overly revealing at other times. We present snapshots of ourselves. We put our best foot forward: a 'whitewashed' version of ourselves. We're connecting, yes, but it's not exactly real.

Have you ever experienced the feeling of being very alone and even lonely in a huge crowd? I certainly have. At times, I crave a deeper, more meaningful connection. I yearn for social intimacy with a fellow human being on the path of awakening, and will often proactively seek out such connection.

Maybe that's why the nerves were creeping in just a bit as I headed downstairs to my interview. On some level, I knew I was stepping into a whole other world – a world of profound connection, of showing up, of being raw and real.

Dr. Lori stood in the lobby, waiting to greet me – her face beaming. Her presence was sweet, kind and gracious. She was beautifully put together, organized and professional. She'd 'staked out' a lovely quiet corner for us. Instantly, I knew I'd stepped out of my confident public speaker shoes and into a new pair of shoes – ones that didn't feel overly familiar, yet were also incredibly comfortable and safe. Almost like slippers.

As you will experience in reading this inspiring book, Dr. Lori quickly becomes like a long lost friend. She listens deeply and profoundly, and elicits deep wells of memories, thoughts and feelings, stories and insights. In holding space for me and others, and then sharing these stories so that we all may become stronger, she shows empathy like nobody I've ever met before.

It takes a willingness to be vulnerable to create this core connection that allows our souls to truly be seen. As vulnerability expert researcher, Dr. Brené Brown states, "Vulnerability is about showing up and being seen. It's tough to do that when we're terrified about what people might see or think." (Hence the reason so many people on Facebook prefer to present an edited version of their lives.)

On my flight back to California that day, I read Dr. Lori's previous book, *Greedy for Life: A Memoir on Aging with Gratitude* from cover to cover. I laughed out loud and was moved to tears many times (I'm sure my seat mate was most puzzled by my behavior), underlining and highlighting key phrases and quotes. As with her new book, *Put on Your Big-Girl Shoes*, Dr. Lori invites you on a journey that feels intimate and personal. We see far more than mere snapshots—we see deeply into the reality of being courageous and claiming your power.

Dr. Lori will take you through multi-sensory, visceral experiences with intellectual insights. Issues of self-doubt, indifference, trauma and fear are revealed through the beautifully told stories of these inspiring women.

This book is full of stories of real women facing real fears, and coming out on the other side stronger, freer and more successful. May you be inspired and empowered to show up and be seen. And, may you, too, have the feeling of being understood at a deep level.

Many blessings
Mari

Mari Smith
Forbes' Top Social Media Power Influencer
Premier Facebook Marketing Expert & Social Media Thought Leader
Author of The New Relationship Marketing and coauthor of Facebook Marketing: An Hour A Day.

Acknowledgments

TO STEP INTO our courage is not a task we can accomplish alone. My deepest gratitude and admiration start with the brave people who shared their personal stories and private thoughts with me so that we can all be inspired to stand up. Rachel Maddow, who despite a ridiculously busy schedule invited an unknown psychologist from Cleveland, Ohio, to her studio for an honest and unfiltered conversation about insecurities: Rachel's sense of humor and welcoming style helped me conquer my own fear of interviewing arguably the smartest interviewer in America. Stefani Schaefer, for the resilient spirit that allowed her to relive the pain of her story so that others could find their own strength to cope with tragedies. Rena Finder, who changed my life: sitting in the presence of this amazing woman forced me to look deeply inside myself to hear the subtle voices of prejudice, indifference, and apathy. I will be forever indebted to her for her courage to step back into a dark place so that the rest of us can become eyewitnesses to the danger of indifference and learn to live a life of honor. Dr. Deborah Plummer, whose story, friendship, and life-long mentorship have helped shape me into the psychologist and person I am today. Margot Stern Strom, Mari Smith, and Andre Parhamovich, who trusted me with their stories and allowed me to share them. Lastly, all of the brave men and women I have had the privilege of professionally counseling over the past two decades, who have taught me about the power of the human spirit.

The book-writing process is not fun or easy—actually it is often downright hard and painful. Thank you, thank you to Katrin Schumann, not only for your brilliant editing skills but for your kind encouragement, which helped me step into my big-girl shoes as a writer. To Ursula DeYoung, for your masterful editing and gentle respect in maintaining my voice. To Trevor Blosser, for your brilliant graphic skills in creating an amazing cover.

Finally, to my 104-year-old Nana. You continue to wear those big-girl shoes with grace and conviction and inspire us all. To my parents, Bill and Joann, who first put those shoes of confidence on my feet and never let me fall: I love you. I am blessed to be a member of a five-generation family that consistently shows up for me, and for that I am eternally grateful. My beautiful daughters, Sarah and Katie, you make this life meaningful. Your compassion for others makes me proud beyond words. May you always stand proud in your big-girl shoes, even when it is hard.

To my husband, Jay, you make all my accomplishments meaningful and all my disappointments insignificant. You are the reason I am able to put the shoes on and live with courage.

"When the whole world is silent, even one voice becomes powerful."

— MALALA YOUSAFZAI

Contents

Introduction

"Give a girl the right pair of shoes, and she can conquer
the world."

— MARILYN MONROE

THERE IS AN ancient Native American proverb that says, "It takes a thousand voices to tell a single story." Our life stories are shaped by our ancestors, cultures, life experiences, and relationships with family and friends. Each of these elements breathes life into our actions and color into our emotions. They are the many voices in our head who whisper our story.

However, unlike fictional or biographical stories, our life stories don't start at the beginning but rather in the middle. After all, the middle is now—the moment that we are standing in. The middle is the tapestry of all that we have woven together from our beginnings, which provided the context for the present we are standing in. The ending of our story is simply the place we are heading toward—the unknown that can be perceived or imagined only by the way we live here in the middle. Walking consciously and deliberately through the moments on our life's journey requires us to step into our grown-up shoes and discover our strength and our resilience.

Every day we weave our life story through our moments on earth: all 87,400 of them. That is roughly how many seconds or moments we are given in a day, our life moments. Moments that are life-changing, but only when we mindfully stand in them. Moments that we savor and cherish, that make us grateful to be alive. Moments that make us vulnerable, the ones filled with intolerable pain that forces us to dig deep into our souls to find a way to breathe, to cope, and to survive. Moments when we listen to the running script in our head of self-doubt and then consciously choose to change the channel and take a risk.

Moments when we make a choice to sit silently and watch injustice occur, or moments when we realize that the stories we are weaving about ourselves and others are fraught with prejudice and so make a moral choice to weave a new story. Moments when we stop looking for information and examples to confirm our biases and prejudices but rather step into our courage to hear a different story, even if it is painful.

Stepping into our big-girl shoes is particularly difficult for women, but this is not because we are inherently weaker or less capable than men. Quite the contrary. At our core we strive for perfection, while being simultaneously sensitive to the evaluation of others. The overarching fear that often holds women back is the fear that stepping up to our greatest challenges will leave us visible and exposed. We will be vulnerable to the evaluation and criticism of others, which in turn will influence how we feel about ourselves.

Life pushes us through these moments, making us transition from one state to the next, and so a metamorphosis occurs. Aging is one of those transitions. It creates the proverbial "one foot in and one foot out" passage to a different state.

The Power of Big-Girl Shoes

Of all the things that we rely on to pass through our rites of passages as we age, our shoes seem the most striking: the power of our shoes. On a practical level, they are designed to provide support for the back, to protect our feet from surfaces, to keep us warm, to keep us cool, to help us run, and to keep us free from injury and infections. Historically, simply owning and wearing shoes was a sign of affluence, as slaves and the poor often did not have them. Symbolically, the removal of shoes can be viewed as a sign of reverence; we remove shoes on holy ground or in spiritual rituals, or simply out of respect when entering somebody's home.

Shoes come in all shapes, sizes, and colors, and therefore they can change the appearance of an outfit and the woman wearing them. Even designers encourage women to transform day attire to evening attire by simply stepping out of their business shoes and into sling-back pumps, transforming the outfit. There seems to be a societal norm about shoes: we all have preconceived ideas about what type of shoe is appropriate for what type of event and what type of person. Shoes have rules and meaning.

Shoes can be an extension of our self-view, reflecting an image of ourselves as playful, sporty, sexy, or professional. Shoes also carry symbolic meaning, as they can represent authority and power but also humility. They represent our journey through life, and particularly, for little girls, they represent the transition from childhood to adulthood. Most women can recall their first pair of high-heeled shoes and how they felt when they slipped them on. Later, shoes represent the shift into senior years, when stylish shoes are replaced by practical, safe ones—yet another shift in our perception of ourselves as we move through life's journey.

According to children's stories, our shoes even hold power. It was Cinderella's glass slipper that ultimately landed her the prince. Dorothy from *The Wizard of Oz* discovered that the power to return home had been with her all along—in her ruby-red slippers.

Finding the courage to put on our big-girl shoes means stepping into our confidence to risk failure, to acknowledge and accept our successes, and to discover the ability to live with gratitude.

When I wrote *Greedy for Life: A Memoir on Aging with Gratitude*, I included a chapter entitled "Growing Up: Making the Big-Girl Shoes Fit." It is this chapter that readers seem to identify with most. Apparently I had hit a universal nerve. The symbolism of making our big-girl shoes fit meant taking on life, coping, achieving, and owning the responsibility of our choices—no easy task.

After the book was released, I received messages from diverse women who shared how healing it was to know that we are all in this together—that even outwardly confident and successful women hear quiet, internal voices of doubt. They began to share their stories, and I had the opportunity to hear the internal conversations they were having with themselves—the battering and doubting words, such as "stupid," "weak," "lazy," "no talent," as well as the healing, empowering ones, such as "courage," "strength," "confidence," and "empathy." These powerful positive words pulled the women I spoke with through tragedy, obstacles, self-doubt, and success-limiting fears.

While the stories that these women shared were unique, the common theme that tied them together was an ongoing challenge to cope, achieve, and live a grateful life despite adversity. Each of the stories supported the theory that a thread of insecurity, doubt, and fear runs through most women. We worry that we are masquerading with an external appearance of grace, confidence, and self-assurance, while inside we feel like imposters. But it is only when we recognize our perceived inadequacies, risk sharing the vulnerable feeling of being "exposed" as a fraud, and acknowledge our true talents, that we find our strength and learn to embrace the active process of living with moral courage. It is then that success follows.

So, although we women often look at each other and think that we are the only ones who suffer from doubt and fear, the truth of the matter is that all over the world grown women are trying to keep their little-girl feet in those confident and successful big-girl shoes.

Success in Life

I set out on a journey to learn and listen from the best of the best on how to step into big-girl shoes and succeed. I was interested in hearing how successful women overcame the feeling of being an imposter, and how they pushed past insecurity and fear to reach the peak of their professions. Instead, what I learned from Rachel Maddow, Margot Stern

Strom, Dr. Deborah Plummer, Stefani Schaefer, and others was how they found the courage to know and embrace their own identities, to build resilience, and to create ways of being moral philosophers so they could live authentic lives. This kind of success went beyond their fame, and their stories revealed a deep connection to gratitude. Finally, Rena Finder and her courage as a Holocaust survivor from Schindler's list made me a witness to the danger of indifference and revealed to me the power that one person can possess to stand up and make a difference.

The themes of survival, perseverance, and gratitude that emerged from these women's stories created a much broader definition of success and resilience. I discovered that the symbol of putting on our big-girl shoes was a developmental journey: we not only need to find the confidence to take a seat at the head of the table in a C-suite office, we also need to put those same shoes on to cope with tragedy and to face the fear of failing. Those metaphorical shoes even helped a woman to survive the horrors of the concentration camps and to build a strong and happy life after those experiences.

The fact that such a diverse group of women could share both fears and strengths reminded me that we are all more similar than different. As women we tend to either put each other on a pedestal—diminishing ourselves in the process—or we put each other down in an attempt to elevate our own self-image. Either way, we create a very narrow perspective, a one-dimensional view that ignores the complexities of being a woman and of being human. It is in all of us both to feel confident and to battle self-doubt, to struggle with tragedies and losses and yet to maintain the capacity to feel joy, to experience the worst of what human beings are capable of and to be touched by the best they have to offer.

This book is not a how-to book about finding your confidence in ten easy steps. Rather, I will take you on a life-changing journey by exploring the complex and vivid stories of other women. I hope that these stories will inform your own choices on how to live. They offer opportunities to eavesdrop on the internal conversations of seemingly very different women, who have all experienced the challenge of making their big-girl

PART I

Facing the Fear, the Self,
and the Imposter

CHAPTER 1

Authenticity: What Do Your Big-Girl Shoes Look Like?

"People are going to realize that I'm a great fraud, and [my career] will end, so I better make sure this is a good show because it'll be my last. Part of me feels that way every day."

— RACHEL MADDOW

THE ROOM WAS dark, with only a crack of light creeping around the edge of the blind. The light flashed red, creating a pulsing image on the bedroom wall that was accompanied by a faint whirling sound. I glanced at the alarm clock: 3:06 am. I knew it was set for 5:00 am, but there would be no more sleep for me. I got up and walked to the window. The red lights were coming from the life-flight helicopter landing pad, which was in clear view from my fifteenth-floor bedroom window. The apartment complex sat in the center of the Henry Ford Hospital complex in Detroit, Michigan. The hospital was massive in size, and from my window it appeared simultaneously beautiful and intimidating.

I stared at the flashing lights, wondering if a life was about to be saved or if it would end on this Tuesday morning in August. While this was perhaps an odd thought to be pondering at such an early hour for a twenty-six-year-old, I knew it was my new reality. I was about to begin my clinical psychology internship. The program offered everything I wanted: it was my first choice, my stretch goal, so when the call came offering me the spot, I cried. I couldn't believe they had selected me. My graduate program was not the strongest in the country, nobody from the school had ever been accepted before, and yet here I was looking down at an amazing hospital and feeling as if I didn't belong. There must have been a mistake. I had left a husband and my comfortable life back in Ohio for this opportunity. The excitement that I felt when the acceptance came seemed years away and was now replaced by tremendous doubt. My eyes moved further down the building to the windows several stories above the Emergency Room doors, where the Intensive Care Units were located. This was where my first day would begin. The thought made me nauseous. I did not feel prepared. I needed more training, more support, and maybe more adult supervision.

The day before, my orientation had consisted of sitting in a large auditorium, gathering binder after binder of useful information about the hospital. We had learned about our rotations from each of our different supervisors, participated in a basic tutorial on the computer system, and collected maps to help us locate the cafeteria, the record room, and the morgue—in that order. None of this information had made me feel emotionally prepared or ready. As I stared out the window, my heart began to race with the thought of what was facing me. I could feel a tear on my cheek. I really just wanted to be waking up with a cup of coffee, kissing my husband good-bye as he left for work, and then calling my grandmother to chat. But that would not be my day today.

The Experience of Shame

I stepped into the shower. I was keenly aware of the importance of dressing in a professional manner—not too casual, not sexy. Still, I would resist those old-lady clothes for as long as I could. I chose an olive-colored dress and my gray pumps with the sensible heels (a message that had been driven into my mind throughout graduate school: heels not too high and not too low, color not too flashy, and style conservative, i.e. boring). I slipped on the freshly pressed white lab coat that had been delivered the night before. It covered most of my dress, and over the left pocket was embroidered "Dr. Lori Stevic-Rust." The butterflies in my stomach returned. I put my pocket-size DSMIII manual (the diagnostic Bible for psychologists) and my laminated card with approved medical abbreviations into my pocket and clipped on my name tag. I was ready—at least that is what it looked like when I glanced in the mirror.

As the elevator door opened, the sterile smell of the Intensive Care Unit hit me. It was a familiar smell from childhood. I pushed the thought aside and stepped onto the floor. I was ready to complete my first consultation on an AIDS patient who was refusing care and asking to die. The lights in the hallway were bright, and the sound of machines beeping seemed to mirror the pounding in my chest. My supervisor was Dr. Richard Portman, an elderly man with gray hair and glasses worn low on the bridge of his nose, making him appear regal. He was a well-respected physician who made interns and residents very nervous. I was certainly no exception. There he sat, waiting for me at the nurses' station. I stepped behind the counter and positioned myself in the swivel seat next to him.

He opened up Room Three's chart and proceeded to walk me through its essential features: the lab section, the consult section, the history and physical, the physician's orders and notes, and finally the nurse's section. I tried desperately to remember all he was saying, but my heart was pounding and my mouth was dry. My nerves were getting the better of me. I had a fleeting thought of asking him for a Valium but thought better of it. He had just met me, and it was still unclear whether or not he had a sense of humor. I knew he was a Pittsburgh Steelers fan, and I found humor in that—being a Browns fan. Thank God Dr. Portman could not hear my thoughts. He rose from the chair, tipping his head and waiting for me to follow him.

At the door, a big red stop sign indicated the need for universal precautions. I quickly stepped into my shoe covers and put on a gown, gloves, and a face mask. The precautions were to protect staff from contracting or spreading infectious diseases and also to protect the patients, whose immune systems were often compromised, from staff bringing infections into the room. The year was 1988; much was still unknown about AIDS, and fear drove many decisions and assumptions. Drugs were being produced and studied, but access was not equitably distributed, and financial limitations precluded many from getting the much-needed drugs. For most of the world, AIDS was "a gay disease" and as such elicited many biases and beliefs that were absent with other conditions. I was keenly aware of the reactions of the more experienced staff, who seemed to manage Room Three differently. Their wariness only contributed to my own apprehension.

This particular case provoked fear in me that reached beyond my inexperience and the normal self-doubt of a first day on a job. While I had read about AIDS and intellectually understood the symptoms and neurological presentations, I had no face to put to the words. I didn't know anybody personally who had the disease, nor had I encountered any patients suffering from the disease before today. I was afraid of what I might see when I walked through the door. Most certainly, I was emotionally unprepared for what I was about to experience.

The room was dimly lit, with the blinds pulled down. The TV was off. There were no flowers, no get-well cards or balloons—just a room with a bed, machines, and a small nightstand. Lying in the bed was a young man only two years older than I was. He was frail and looked much older than his stated age. (That's how we describe people in the world of healthcare. I guess it means we have a benchmark for how we think people at certain ages should look.) He was connected to many different machines, and tubes were coming from all parts of his body. I imagine he felt as well as looked a lifetime older than his stated age. I tried to avoid taking in the scene as a whole, for it increased the feeling of nausea that I had been struggling with since I'd gotten out of bed.

As I slowly approached his bed, I glanced at this arms, which were covered in dark purple, raised lesions called Kaposi's sarcoma. This type of cancer is often seen in AIDS patients and causes patches of abnormal tissue to grow on the internal organs, mouth, and nose, as well as under the skin.

He looked up at me. His eyes were a brilliant shade of blue but had sunk so deep that they looked lost and distant. He was thin and frail and appeared to be laboring to breathe; the same lesions that were on his skin were also present in his lungs. As I got closer to the bed, I noticed that he was slowly moving his arms under the sheets in an attempt to hide their appearance.

I glanced past the bed to his nightstand. There was a water glass with a straw and a picture in a wooden frame. The picture showed two young men, smiling, with leafy trees and bicycles in the background. He noticed my glance and said, "Yes. That used to be me." I was embarrassed by his words because it is was in fact what I had been wondering. The young man to the left was handsome, with thick wavy hair, a muscular frame, and deep blue eyes. Physically there appeared to be only remnants of that person lying in the bed.

I introduced myself and asked if I could put some questions to him. I found myself focusing on those deep blue eyes; it was striking how much they revealed about him. They seemed to be screaming, "I am still a person!" But his voice could muster only weak-sounding, defeated words. He suggested that I might want to step further back from his bed. In that moment, I wondered what I must look like to him—covered from head to toe in protective gear and talking to him through a mask. Maybe he sensed my fear, or maybe he was used to feeling and being treated like a leper. There was so much shame in that room: my shame about my own fear and thoughts, his shame about his condition, his appearance, the circulating belief that he was gay and had "done this to himself." The world then seemed emotionally distant and personally removed from the "gay disease." There was a common view in our country that AIDS was God's punishment for those who were gay. And these views were not lost on the young man lying in the bed, covered with sores and shame.

I felt too inexperienced to understand this man's decision to stop treatment and die. I wanted so badly to understand his depression and despair, but what could I possibly know about being treated as a leper, lying alone in a hospital room, waiting to die, with no family sitting outside because they had disowned him years ago? A deep sadness washed over me. This young man needed an experienced professional to help him navigate the painful life-and-death decisions that he was struggling to make. Unfortunately, what he got was a new intern on her first day, who had no idea where to begin.

I went through the motions of what I thought was expected of me, but I felt overwhelmed and lost. I could not hold back my tears. Excusing myself, I left the room. I stood in the hallway, feeling inadequate, lost, ashamed, scared, and sad about the realities that I would have to face to work in this profession. My tears were freely flowing. This was not how I wanted my supervisor to see me. It was not how a professional in big-girl shoes was supposed to behave. And it certainly was not how I wanted to see myself.

In that moment I realized I had two choices: I could pull myself together because psychologists don't cry, or so I had been taught—or I could go back into that room and allow the patient to see the insecurity I was feeling and hear the shuffling sound of my ill-fitting big-girl shoes.

When I pushed the door open and stepped back inside, the young man lying in the bed turned and looked at me. I pulled up a chair and moved closer to the bed, and for the next hour I listened to him talk, cry, and share his fears. I told him mine. As I stood to leave the room, he thanked me for really listening and for not pretending to fully understand his circumstances. He thanked me for "being a real doctor." "You know," he added, "for not faking it."

That compliment stuck to me like a piece of Velcro. I realized in that moment that what he saw in me was the very strength I saw in myself but often doubted; he saw my reason for wanting to be a psychologist in the first place.

While this experience took place more than twenty-eight years ago, what I learned about courage that day framed my professional and personal life. I developed a deep understanding of the power of courage. The courage to really examine the image I held of myself—my thoughts, my beliefs, my internal view of who I am. I was so focused that day on feeling like an imposter that I almost became one. I almost became the psychologist I thought I was expected to be: the serious, technical scientist, who intellectually understood emotional struggles but didn't feel them, who could diagnose and treat but was afraid to empathize. On closer examination, however, I found that I was really a young woman, an untested psychologist, a serious scientist who also had a sense of humor, a professional who could be moved to tears, a woman who wore high heels and a white coat, an inexperienced doctor who had much to learn but already possessed the capacity to connect with people in her own, unscripted, and unique way. This style had often been criticized and reviled by supervisors in my graduate school because it brought in "too much of my personality" when working with patients. But that day, at Henry Ford Hospital in the hallway outside Room Three, I experienced the power of authenticity.

Researchers describe this kind of authenticity as "the courage to be imperfect." It requires the active choice of letting go of our expectations of who we should be and choosing instead to be who we really are. Letting go of the imposter we hold inside gives us the freedom to embrace our limitations and strengths. When I stopped pretending and became "real," that day in Room Three, I discovered the power of human connection.

Over the next several months, I saw Nelson, the young man in Room Three, regularly. He had a life story, as we all do, and hearing it changed me. He stopped being "Room Three with AIDS" and became a person with a terminal disease. As a clinician, I learned to see the disease through the eyes of the person it afflicted. Nelson informed my style as a new psychologist in a way that ten years of training had not been able to do. He gave me permission to be myself, with all my flaws and strengths. When I stepped into my authentic shoes, I discovered compassionate courage.

Nelson died just before Halloween that year. I remember it well: the sterilization of his empty room and the shrugs of the staff, who had long since emotionally disconnected from him. But mostly I remember him. The young man who felt so ashamed and meaningless, who was invisible to so many, taught me about the power of being seen, of human connection, and the art of unfiltered listening. He taught me to be a "real psychologist."

The concept of being "real"—genuine and true to our own image and beliefs about ourselves—is often created early and then shaped and

The more authentic and real our self-image is, the more it is able to absorb feedback from others that is consistent, while discounting or challenging feedback that is inconsistent. An honest evaluation of the self requires the acknowledgment and acceptance of gifts and weaknesses, both of which are necessary for balance. To seek perfection may, in essence, remove us from our own humanity and thus make us self-focused and preoccupied. If we are so busy looking at ourselves, how can we ever be emotionally available to see others?

If we can't slip our feet into the shoes of confidence and clear identity, we live in fear. Fear of being seen. Fear of failing. Fear of evaluation. Fear of being foolish. Fear of being "caught" as the imposter that our insecurity tells us we are. For successful women, the stakes get higher: leaders are often more visible than others, as being seen is part of the image and role of a leader. The problem is that women who are visible and successful are often seen by others only through the lens of success. They become one-dimensional. Perhaps we as women not only feel like imposters when we distort our own self-view but create the imposters in each other when we hold other women to a one-dimensional standard.

This seems to be particularly true when we look at famous, successful women and then compare ourselves to them. What if we could know the complexity of these women, their weaknesses and fears coupled with their strengths and talents, and only then compare ourselves? One such highly visible woman, Rachel Maddow, offers a fascinating insight into what can happen when we step into our big-girl shoes, embracing our complexities fully.

Walking through Insecurity and Fear

As the car pulled up to the entrance of the NBC Studio at 30 Rockefeller Center in New York City, my heart started to beat faster. I pushed open the door and stepped onto the green marble floor with the words "30 Rockefeller" embedded in gold. I was escorted to the registration area, where my photo was taken and an ID created so I could pass through security.

The studio seemed much smaller than it appears on television. The back wall was illuminated with the familiar "Rachel Maddow Show" images. The desk was a small half-moon with one chair. There were three cameras and two large-screen TV sets, used for viewing the b-roll, or footage shown to the audience during the show, as well as the shots of any guests being interviewed remotely. A black curtain separated the studio from the many cubicles of the staff-members, who were moving quickly back and forth from their computers to the studio. Some were speaking into headsets, others were printing materials and rushing to place them in their appropriate spots.

Kelsey, Rachel's assistant, had placed a swivel chair for me along the curtained wall. The cameraman approached and gave me an earpiece so I could hear the entire show. The studio was quiet, and I tried to take in the scene. I reached into my purse and for the third time checked that my phone was turned off.

It had been only a few weeks since the message arrived that Rachel had agreed to my request to interview her about her big-girl shoes. This was my biggest reach—my long-shot request. And when she actually agreed, it became my biggest fear. I was about to step completely out of my comfort zone to interview Rachel Maddow. My one-dimensional view of Rachel was as a woman with confidence: secure in herself, bold, intellectually razor-sharp, fearless, and famous. This view was reflected in the reactions I received from many of my friends and colleagues, who wondered how talking to her could possibly be helpful in learning about the concepts of insecurity and fear. In fact, even Rachel's staff seemed confused as to why I was reaching out to her to talk about these concepts. But I had thought that if a famous, successful woman of great confidence could give us a glimpse into her own fears as well as her courage, we could learn something about the power of authenticity.

As soon as the email arrived with the final approval of details and time, I began to prepare. The truth is that I instantly started to panic: What had I been thinking? Everybody had suggestions for what questions I should ask. Even my 103-year-old grandmother got in on the action and gave me advice about what shoes I should wear. Nana had been listening to me for weeks as I shared with her every interesting fact that I uncovered about Rachel—including the fact that she always carries a handkerchief in her pocket. By her own admission, Rachel is sentimental and can often be moved to tears, so she keeps the handkerchief handy. She is also a bit superstitious, and once the hanky is settled in a certain pocket it must remain there for the duration. As I packed my bags the night before, Nana had asked me to go into her cedar chest and take out one of her original handkerchiefs, edged with old lace and embroidery, to give to Rachel as a thank-you gift from her. And, true to her sentimental side, Rachel did become emotional when I presented this gift to her.

During my three weeks of preparation, I watched countless hours of Rachel being interviewed—by David Letterman, Meet the Press, Jay Leno, Howard Stern, Jon Stewart, Jimmy Fallon, Ellen DeGeneres. Each of them offered more background information. I even managed to dig up and read Rachel's undergraduate Stanford thesis, "Identifiable Lives: AIDS and the Response to Dehumanization." I felt ready when I boarded the plane bound for LaGuardia airport.

But as I sat alone in her quiet studio, the buzz in my head grew louder. I was recalling phrases used by seasoned and famous interviewers: "smartest woman," "articulate and fiercely prepared," and my favorite, "intimidated by her intellect." Here I was, not a reporter, not a journalist, and really not even a writer, just a psychologist from Cleveland, Ohio, waiting in the MSNBC studio in New York City to interview Her. My thoughts were interrupted—thank God—by some activity in the studio.

The staff and crew were hustling about. The large digital clock read 8:47 pm. There were exactly thirteen minutes to live television. A young woman entered the studio and placed a red coffee mug with the words "Rachel Maddow" on the desk, along with a stack of papers, and then disappeared behind the curtain. The clock advanced to 8:55, and the camera crew moved into place. Another woman entered from the back wall and took her place on the platform next to Rachel's chair, make-up kit in hand. I thought, "Something must be wrong, there are only three minutes until the live broadcast." Just then, at 8:57, Rachel came bounding into the studio from an open curtain to the left. She moved with quick, bouncing steps onto the platform. She was wearing black tennis shoes and her signature Levi jeans, a purple cotton shirt, and a black suit jacket.

She took her seat at the desk and pulled her jacket away from her neck, allowing the make-up artist to brush powder on her face and neck while the camera crew snaked the cord for her earpiece and microphone up through her jacket. She made no eye contact with anybody. The clock read 8:58 as the crew rushed off set. Rachel buttoned her jacket, pulled her chair closer to the desk, and typed quickly on her keypad without looking up. A crew-member began the countdown: thirty seconds, camera two. Five, four, three, two… Without missing a beat, Rachel looked up into the camera, flashed a smile, and with great interest and enthusiasm began her discussion with the viewers.

She was animated and conversational, providing insight and information with humor, energy, and style. Her lead story was about the interesting things happening in Oregon—including a government official who was asking citizens to mail him urine specimens for his research on aging, and a story of owls attacking joggers. There were segments on Rand Paul and his beliefs about vaccines, and updates on policy issues and ISIS. During each commercial break, she remained laser-focused. She spoke quietly into her earpiece on a few occasions, typed and changed copy, and shaved time off segments. Her attention and concentration was so intense that she appeared to be unaware of anybody else or anything going on in the studio. I, on the other hand, was keenly aware of everything, particularly my growing anxiety. I worried that I might be a distraction, sitting in a chair only ten feet from her desk. I worried that I was in her line of vision when she was looking into camera number two and interviewing her guests. But by the third commercial break, it had become very clear that she was free from distractions. Her intense focus was on actively listening to her guests and delivering the content she had prepared. She didn't see or notice any of us around her.

The hour flew by. Eventually she gave a gentle salute and signed off to the upcoming show, and with that The Rachel Maddow Show came to an end. The hustle and movement in the studio began again as the set was dismantled and the crew moved about, attending to the cameras and papers left on the desk. I stood up and removed my earpiece, handing it to one of the staff-members as she approached.

Bouncing off the set with a warm smile and her hand extended, Rachel greeted me. "You must be Dr. Lori," she said. We talked briefly about our interview the next day, and she asked if she needed to do any "homework ahead of time." I immediately felt relaxed. We took a few selfie photos and laughed as I assured her that I had done enough homework for the both of us. Then she hugged me good-bye and quickly left the studio. It wasn't until I was back on the first floor near the NBC studio entrance on 45th street, waiting for my driver, that the reality fully hit me: I was going to have lunch and a conversation with Rachel Maddow.

Taking the First Tentative Steps

I sat at the table near the window, looking out at the ice-skaters on the rink at Rockefeller plaza. The sun was shining through the flags and glistening off the ice. I had arrived fifteen minutes—okay, an hour early for our lunch. I took out my audio recorder, a few pages of typed notes, and my glasses. Then I sat back and took a deep breath, glancing under the table at my striped purple, gray, and black pumps. Yep, I did in fact have on my big-girl shoes, and I was ready to interview arguably the smartest interviewer and one of the most successful women on television.

With the same bouncing strides that I had seen the night before, Rachel entered the restaurant and approached the table. She greeted me with a hug and sat down. We exchanged some personal stories, ordered lunch, turned the tape recorder on, and began the interview. Without looking at my notes or following the sequence of questions I had prepared, I asked about her early years as an AIDS activist and how it had influenced her young identity.

She sat back in her seat, took a deep breath, and stared out the window. I began to worry that I had perhaps offended her or crossed the line with my first question. Was the interview going to come to an end before it even got started? After what felt like a very long silence, she leaned forward. Looking me directly in the eye, she smiled and said in a quiet voice, "My preface on this is to say I don't usually talk about these things—this is more touchy-feely than I usually allow myself to be—so I probably won't have a great vocabulary for this."

She was wrong. She did in fact have a great vocabulary, and for the next several hours we talked. Her honesty, vulnerability, sense of humor, and incredible spirit led the way.

Around the same time that I had been learning about AIDS and sitting with those who carried the virus and the stigma, Rachel Maddow had made a place for herself in the front row. At seventeen, two important truths were stirring inside her: "I'm gay, and my people are dying." This was her first conscious integration of her own identity with the marginalized community. She was a senior in high school, a time when most girls are focused on the lighter side of teenage life. Rachel was secretly volunteering at the Center for AIDS Service in Oakland, California, near her home. There she gained a graphic and personal view of death and of the indifference of all around her concerning this supposedly "gay disease."

It was the late eighties, and the AIDS epidemic was at its peak. AZT drugs had just come on the market, and, while they helped a little, their distribution and cost prevented them from reaching many. Rachel remembers thinking, "If this is true about me—that I am gay—then I am a part of this battle for survival." At times the battle was militant, a fierce effort to "save ourselves because the rest of the world didn't care about us." She added, "I so desperately wanted to be useful."

These two realities—AIDS and injustice—formed her world alongside her typical high-school life, which was filled with sports and healthy friends, prom dresses and acceptance into college. This dual and often disconnected image was her internal view of herself, the self that is created from a variety of sources, including perceptions, life experiences, and the feedback we get from others.

Our gender, sexuality, race, and ethnicity are things we usually know about ourselves. Then there are the pieces that float around us until we grapple with them and decide which concepts to pull in and which ones to reject. Am I fat? Am I pretty? Am I strong? Am I a follower? Am I artistic? Am I athletic? Am I smart? Am I shy? Do people like me? Do people fear me? Do I believe in God? What do I believe about differences in people? What is my purpose? How do I feel about poverty? What is my responsibility in fighting social injustice?

All of these questions float in and out of our conscious awareness as we attempt the integration process. The acceptance and rejection of particular notions about ourselves is how we create an identity. Then we learn to incorporate both negative and positive feedback from others and weave that into the views we already hold. This integration is fundamental in the shaping and adjusting of our self-concept and the esteem or value we place in ourselves.

A consistent shared view between the image of ourselves expressed by the outside world and the image we create for our internal self leads to confidence and courage and minimizes fear. But first the internal view needs to be fully formed. Rachel's internal battle consciously began during her early years in high school. She was an athlete, taking part in volleyball, basketball, and swimming. In our interview she laughed and said, "But not softball as you might have thought." She competed well in each of the sports and was a social person, engaged with her teammates. But internally she was a self-described introvert, battling her own issues of doubt.

She dated throughout high school, but never just one person. "Even when I thought I was heterosexual, I never imagined myself tied to just one person," she said. In fact, she wasn't even a serial monogamist during her dating years. She never had fantasies of marriage, having children, or being paired with one person for the rest of her life. She felt disconnected from the feelings and conversations of her friends on these issues. Instead she was struggling with her own private analysis and questions about herself. This struggle was emotional, of course, but, in a style consistent with her strength of intellect, she began to reason her way through her internal turmoil. By the age of seventeen, she had "figured out" through her own deductive reasoning that she was gay. This realization gave her both peace and torment. She knew that sharing this information and coming out in her very conservative town would not be safe for her.

Already Rachel knew social injustice at a deep level and felt passionate about working to make a difference. Her spirit and conviction are evident in her high-school commencement address. That windy day in May, she approached the podium wearing her Birkenstock shoes and knee-high white socks, her yellow gown whipping open with every gust of wind. She placed a white sheet of paper on the podium, took off her square cap, and placed it on the shelf under the podium.

In front of her was the Castro Valley graduating class of 1990. The program said that she would give a speech entitled, "What a Long Strange Trip It Has Been," but instead, she explained, she had decided to "say the things that I wanted to say over the past four years." The five teachers sitting behind her, facing the audience, squirmed a bit in their seats, and the two on the end glanced at each other, anticipating her "off-script" speech.

With her long blonde hair and dangling gold earrings flying in the wind, Rachel opened with a pronouncement: "We no longer have to let society happen to us, we get to create our own." She commented that the "upper-middle-class community that is Castro Valley, while nestled in one of the most politically and culturally diverse areas of the nation, is filled with many leaders, parents, and teachers who are closed-minded and afraid to allow change to happen." The crowd roared and clapped when she added that, despite the diversity that surrounded them, "their parents and leaders can't even say 'condom' in front of each other." Rachel ended by imploring her high-school classmates to give something back to the community: "Don't assume that things won't change. Make them change." The crowd clapped and cheered as she walked down the ramp off the platform. Through the applause, the woman doing the amateur taping can be heard saying, "One day she is going to do something wonderful."

This young blonde with showy earrings may not resemble the Rachel Maddow who is followed by millions today, but her message is the same: "Strive to become the best you can be about the things you are most passionate about." Yet, when she thinks about herself at that age, Rachel sees and hears a self-indulgent kid filled with attitude. It makes her uncomfortable.

Shedding the Imposter

A decision about college had to be made. While there is a laser-sharp focus and strategic quality to Rachel today, at age seventeen she was more casual about life decisions. In fact, her application to Yale was sent in two weeks after the deadline. Her fleeting thought was, "Maybe they won't notice or care." Her other applications were sent to schools that offered her volleyball scholarships and then to Stanford because—well, it was far from home.

She thinks of her acceptance to Stanford as a "lark of the universe." Rachel laughed as she shared that she was the 1,596th student accepted out of 1,600 students. The majority of the admission officers were men who were not impressed with her application, but there was one woman on the committee who lobbied for her admission. It was Rachel's compelling essay and role as an activist that this woman highlighted. She felt that Rachel could be a significant political force on the campus. "I knew it was a fluke that I was accepted, but I don't think they regret accepting me," Rachel added with a smile.

Stanford University is located in the heart of Silicon Valley, between San Francisco and San Jose, on eight thousand acres of rolling hills. Once she'd arrived on the campus, it didn't take Rachel long to realize that the inline-skating, email-corresponding, world-traveled girls who shared her all-girls dorm were nothing like her. The majority of them were focused and driven, with their majors already decided. "They were going to be the neurosurgeon like their father and his father. The practice was waiting for them when they graduated," she said, laughing.

In stark contrast, Rachel arrived on the campus without a single idea for a major or an academic direction. And that wasn't the only difference she felt. She laughed again and confessed that prior to college, "I had never even had Chinese food or knew anybody who had been out of the country, or for that matter anyone who even had a passport." Yet there she was, a freshman at one of the most prestigious schools in the country. The thought that she was there on a lark was academically liberating, as it gave her the freedom to explore classes that were simply of interest to her. However, on the social side, her disconnection from her peers soon began to create great stress. For one thing, it was becoming increasingly difficult to hide and ignore her sexual identity.

Her strategy for coping with this disconnection was to take on homophobic comments boldly and directly. She wanted to put a face to the words being used, but she admits that she was afraid of the consequences. So one day when she was sick with the flu, in what she called an "immature and self-focused gesture," she climbed out of bed and marched to the dorm restroom. Maybe she was delirious from the flu, or maybe the anxiety was getting to her, but she had convinced herself that it would be easier to tackle the issue head-on. She could not tolerate her mounting anxiety about being closeted. Her solution was to tape a note in the bathroom of Paloma, her freshman college dorm. The note essentially announced that yes, she was gay, "so get over it." She smiled as she told me this and took another bite of her sandwich. "I was seventeen but acting like I was fourteen, in the way that I came out," she said. And it gets worse.

Rachel was one of only two freshmen on the Stanford campus who were openly gay, which made her admission newsworthy. The headline of the Stanford Daily read, "Freshmen Lesbians Face Coming Out with Fear, Relief." The paper interviewed Rachel, who shared that she felt supported by her friends and relieved not to be keeping her orientation a secret any longer. The article went on to say, "The only people whom Maddow has not informed are her parents. Seeing no urgent need to tell them, she said she has decided to wait on it." This is one of Rachel's biggest regrets as she looks back. Shortly before the article was published, Rachel had decided to go home and tell her parents. Unfortunately, the article ran and somebody mailed a copy to them before she could get there.

Rachel sighed. "They did not know how to handle it. It was a terrible time for all of us." Her parents are devout Catholics, and in their bewilderment they disowned her. She found herself truly on her own. She doesn't blame them or hold any animosity toward them; instead, she empathizes with them. "I was so rude and uncaring in the way I handled this. I think they could not believe that they had raised such an uncaring and callous daughter. I was selfish in the way I came out." The painful separation that lasted for the next several years did yield one benefit: it allowed her and her parents to "start from ground zero and rebuild a relationship." Her mother is now her best friend and confidant, her father her "coach and buddy." But the rebuilding process required all of them to reconstruct how they viewed themselves and each other, which was no easy task.

Insecurity and doubt arise when the themes and fundamental plot of our life stories are not consistent or able to hold together. Sometimes this occurs when the way we feel on the inside—that internal Velcro strip of our created identity, which holds onto feedback from others—is significantly different from the feedback we receive from the outside world. Similarly, when trauma disrupts our self-concept and we are forced to rearrange our internal view, we may experience an uncomfortable disconnect—for example, when a father who has lost his daughter in Iraq searches to reconstruct his internal view of himself, as a man who is no longer her father, and struggles to find meaning in a life without his child (for more on this story, see Chapter 6).

Disconnections of this kind shake our confidence and lie at the core of the "imposter" feeling—the all-too-familiar notion that others will soon discover that their view of us is not really who we are. But often the image we hold on the inside is actually the distorted one. We have the power to create an image of ourselves as not being worthy or adequate, and this distortion blocks us from receiving compliments and positive support— we reject them because they have no place to stick internally.

When I asked Rachel how she viewed herself, she answered that she is the "unlikely one"—the "unlikely Rhodes Scholar, the unlikely kid who got into Stanford, the unlikely woman on television." She seemed confident in her own view of herself but was quick to discount those of others when they seemed inaccurate to her. When I told her that she has been described as one of the country's smartest women, easily intimidating those who interview her or are interviewed by her, she laughed hard. "I have super powers. I can create the impression of being smart and interesting." In a more serious tone, she went on to say that her internal view is that she works really, really hard and puts in tremendous hours of work for the show. She smiled and explained, "If you said I was one of the hardest-working women, I can accept that, but not really the smartest—that doesn't fit."

Consider that Meryl Streep, the actor nominated for more Academy Awards and Golden Globes than any other actor in history, was quoted as saying, "You think, why would anyone want to see me again in a movie? And I don't know how to act anyway, so why am I doing this?" The real question for Meryl is "Can you act? Do you believe that you have a talent for acting?" If the answer is no, then she should stop acting and learn a new skill. But if the answer is yes, then a period should be put at the end of this sentence: "I know I can act."

It is a different question to ask, "Can I learn more and aspire to be an even better actor?" That is not a question about a woman's view of herself but rather a question about the drive to be better, learn more, and improve. It is not a question that sets us up to feel like an imposter. The question that gets to the core of Meryl Streep is the one expressing her doubt about her own skills and thereby her reliance on others to decide whether or not she can act.

This reliance on the views of others over our own sets us up for fear and doubt, because the opinions of others create constantly changing standards that we will never fully satisfy. If, on the other hand, we hold our own view firmly in place, we have a better chance of feeling confident and connected to our identity and to feedback from others. Doing so involves a life-long process of practicing the art of being authentic—with the good, the bad, and the ugly parts fully exposed.

world-renowned authority in vocational guidance, was the instructor. He was a serious-looking professor with a soft demeanor, and his teaching style clearly revealed his passion for the topic. For the life of me, I couldn't imagine why he was so invested in this mission. (How smart and insightful I was at twenty-two years old!)

Yet here I am, all these years later, talking and writing about a phrase—actually a concept—that he first introduced to me. Over the years I have used this concept in therapy, in life, in talks, and in my writing. It is the notion that we "actively master what we passively suffer," that each of us is composed of our obstacles, struggles, and inadequacies, which we consciously or subconsciously spend a lifetime actively mastering or conquering. In other words, we strive to excel at the very thing that makes us feel weak or inadequate, which allows us to use those skills to make social contributions. Thus the individual who casts herself as shy becomes an actress, and the person with a speech impediment becomes a reporter or public speaker. Of course, these are obvious and oversimplified examples. What about those who struggle with a lack of confidence, fears, or insecurities—those who feel powerless and insignificant or are simply searching for a way to feel useful? How do they actively master and overcome these obstacles? For this book, I wanted to understand how women create and accept their self-images, and how they push through fear and pain to step into their big-girl shoes and wear them through life, no matter what it takes. I wanted to figure out how women choose and use work to master their struggles and then make valuable contributions to society.

Back in graduate school, that career-counseling class was just a course I needed to get through before I could get on with the good stuff. But it was in Dr. Savickas's class that I found clarity about myself and my chosen profession. It enabled me to fully understand and shape my self-identity and then to design my life path—and it is probably because of this class that I first rejected the idea of the work/life balance. Working in whatever form we choose—paid or otherwise—is our expression of the self and our sharing of our mastery over our inadequacies or pain, and this is what creates the contribution we ultimately make to others. Work and life are really not separate concepts that we should be battling to balance. Instead we should strive to integrate our work and our personal selves— learning what our strengths are and then using them to push through obstacles and weaknesses to create lasting success.

A Turning Point

Dr. Savickas's office was at the Northeast Ohio Medical University (NEOMED), where he served as the Chair of the Behavioral Science Department—when he wasn't in Portugal, Belgium, South Africa, and the United Kingdom, working as a visiting professor and serving on the editorial boards of twenty-two scholarly journals around the world. He looked and behaved like a real academic professor, with a graying beard and round glasses. He had a gentle and thought-provoking style, and he clearly loved teaching.

In addition to teaching the career courses, Dr. Savickas was actively involved in training medical students in the art of interviewing and behavioral health. As psychology graduate students, we were often invited to come to his office and participate in teaching these courses, a task that I really enjoyed. The added bonus was that his office was just down the hall from the anatomy and physiology labs, and occasionally we were allowed to sit in and observe the dissection of the brain—now that was interesting stuff! But, unfortunately, the career-counseling class was not held at the medical school; it was offered on the KSU campus in one of the old, run-down buildings—a boring topic in a boring place.

The only advantage that I could see to the course was that my dear friends Janet Dix and Beverly Donovan were in the class. They were fourteen years older than I was, wiser and more mature, and they had their nurturing, mothering behavior down to a science. The class was held in the late afternoon, a time that made paying attention hard, which is why Janet and Bev usually came prepared with "snacks" for the class. But not the kind of snacks I often had in my purse—gummy bears and chocolate. They brought grown-up snacks. Bev would arrive with her wooden cutting-board and fancy cheese-cutter, a tool that I didn't even know existed at the time, since the cheese in my refrigerator was already sliced and wrapped in individual plastic. As if we were having some high-end, fancy party, she would slice a variety of cheeses, place fancy-looking crackers (not saltines) alongside the cheeses, and then garnish the arrangement with grapes. She and Janet tell me today that they used food as a lure to keep me coming to class and paying attention. It worked.

Most people think of psychologists as loving and actively engaging in the "touchy-feely" stuff and speaking in "psychobabble," but I wasn't one of those. In fact, I tried my best to avoid self-exploration exercises and usually didn't do well with the "How does that make you feel?" interviewing technique. So, when I read on the career-counseling syllabus that we were going to engage in an "interactive" exercise to explore our life themes by using personal narratives, I conjured up every reason I could to skip class—despite the cheese. As fate would have it, however, I chose to go to class after all, without knowing that the experience would reveal and focus my life—and that thirty years later I would still carry what I learned that day with me.

As I entered the classroom, feeling a bit impatient, I reminded myself that this was just one more hurdle I had to get over. I grabbed a handful of grapes and took my seat. On top of each of our desks was a small booklet with questions that we were instructed to ponder and then answer in vivid and clear form. I skimmed through the pages, reading each of the questions—our earliest recollections, role models, hobbies, favorite books and sayings. Dr. Savickas reminded us that the value in the exercise was not so much in the factual components of our memories but in our interpretation and active rehearsal of those memories—that is what guides our integration of how we view ourselves. With a mixture of anxiety and annoyance, I began to work on the assignment. I stared at the paper in front of me as I recalled one of my earliest memories. I rejected it several times and went searching for a different one, but it continued to be the loudest one in my head. So I began to put the image on paper.

I was lying on a cold examining table, with bright, cruel lights shining on me. I was screaming and crying for my parents, who were forbidden entry into the room. I did not understand what was happening to me. There were adult faces staring down at my four- or five-year-old self. They were hurting me and holding me down. The attempts to catheterize me were not going well, and with each probe I screamed louder. They held me down harder, pinning my legs. They didn't seem to care that I was crying. With my one free hand, I began pulling on my hair; the pain and anxiety were more than I could bear. I screamed, and they continued to try to place the catheter into my bladder. When my parents were finally allowed to enter the room, they found me covered in sweat, my eyes swollen from crying, and a big bald spot on my head. Lying on the table was the pile of hair I had pulled out.

It is an awful memory, and I hate that it is the one that comes to me when I'm asked about my earliest active memories. I had a wonderful childhood, filled with ice cream, movies, loving parents, and friends. But this incident left a wound. As a child I struggled with several medical conditions that often led me back to hospitals and medical facilities. I learned to hate the smell of antiseptic soap, fluorescent lights, and white lab coats. That is until I met Dr. Theresa, who was beautiful and kind and made me laugh. She had long blonde hair and smelled like baby powder, and she was the first doctor who sat next to me, looked me in the eyes, and talked to me. It was Dr. Theresa who brought me an orange Popsicle and showed me the catheter tube and explained where she had to put it. She was the one who made me laugh and then told me to hold my laugh while the tube slipped gently into my bladder. She was the one who softly stroked my hair and told me I was brave. She was the first person to suggest an association between a white coat and kindness. As a graduate student, filling out Dr. Savickas's questionnaire, I stared at my handwritten recollection and began to understand what my professor was trying to tell me.

The next part of the assignment was to identify a few of our heroes or role models and then use adjectives to describe them. The identification of our heroes—not our parents—is the identification of the attributes that we use as a blueprint for our self-construction. I identified Dr. Theresa and described her as compassionate, smart, and funny. Sister Phyllis Marie, one of my high-school teachers, I identified as funny, a selfless giver of knowledge and guidance, and an advocate. This portion of the assignment ended with using the role-model adjectives to describe and inform ourselves. We had to complete the sentence "I am a person who…" by plugging in the adjectives we had used for our heroes. When I put it together, my sentence read, "I am a person who is funny, compassionate, and smart, who uses knowledge to advocate for others."

The next section asked us to list our favorite books. We cognitively script our life journey through the books we read, and more specifically through our favorite parts of the books, which reflect a strategy that we believe will guide us in life. We are drawn to these books and stories because they reflect themes that we connect with and offer an implicit plan to guide us through our life story. My favorite book as a child was *The Velveteen Rabbit* by Margery Williams, which explored authenticity, the power of love, and the painful journey of becoming Real. During my early college years, I was drawn to Maya Angelou's book *I Know Why the Caged Bird Sings*, which tackles the battle to preserve dignity, self-pride, identity, and courage.

Finally, we were instructed to write down our favorite motto or saying. This was the eavesdropping portion of the exercise; we needed to listen to the quiet, internal advice that we give ourselves. I wrote the following: "The two most important days in your life are the day you were born and the day you figure out why," by Mark Twain, and "Courage is about perseverance, not bravery. Be courageous despite the fear," by Maya Angelou.

The completion of this assignment was not a lesson in career guidance but a road map for my life journey. In reading what I had written for the assignment from beginning to end, I saw my life story evolve. I was not in the field of healthcare by accident. I had suffered pain, fear, and confusion as an ill child in a system where I felt unseen. Dr. Theresa had showed me the power of compassion and the art of healing. I learned to actively master my fear of illness, my suffering, and my vulnerability and to turn these weaknesses into the courage to advocate and to heal with compassion. This is how my pain and suffering were converted into a social contribution. I rehearsed the integration of my work and life, which co-mingle to create purpose, by "discovering why I am here and using courage to achieve it."

Turning Meaninglessness into Meaning

When I presented the concept of actively mastering what we passively suffer to Rachel Maddow, she grimaced at the word "suffer." She didn't feel, given all the good that she has in her life—a great relationship, an amazing job, and a loving family—that she should complain or talk about suffering. So I reframed the question as an inquiry into her early obstacles and struggles. Now she was engaged. I took a big swig of my iced tea and asked about her struggle with depression.

She looked out the window at the skaters and thought for a moment. "It's like a fog sweeps over me. I lose my sense of smell, and my taste becomes metallic, and I put on my seatbelt and prepare for the feeling that follows," she said. She paused for another minute. "I suppose it's related to a feeling of sadness, but mostly it feels like a disconnection from meaning. Like there is nothing to compare things to, as nothing in and of itself has meaning. You are just at loose ends in the universe, with no horizon to anchor yourself." Her tattoo of a compass rose serves as a reminder that she has direction and context in the world and that the direction will anchor her to the horizon. It is where hope and safety resides, and it helps her ride the storm of her depression until it passes.

Rachel's active mastery of this struggle is reflected in her mission statement, or guiding principle, for her TV show: to increase the amount of useful information in the world. "I explain the news, and as such I am consistently trying to give meaning to things," she said. Because she knows what meaninglessness can feel like, Rachel orients and actively works on overcoming her depression through meaningful connections.

This is in part how she "builds a life around it." As is the case for many people who battle depression, she often requires strong support to pull through the darkness. Rachel credits her partner, Susan, with being that anchor. When a surge of depression occurs, Rachel can often hear words of hope only from Susan. "She will say to me, 'This is that thing, and it won't last'—I can hear it from her," Rachel explained.

Rachel identified activists—people who act on what they believe—as her role models or heroes. She herself served as an activist for ten years. Instead of joining her fellow students at Stanford in skating, socializing, and emailing, Rachel conducted HIV-training workshops for her peers and ran Ye Olde Safer Sex Shoppe on campus. She told me with a laugh, "It was like doing stand-up comedy as I knocked on doors in the dorms, passing out condoms."

Rachel was living in the height of the HIV/AIDS epidemic, and as a gay student she understood the alienation felt by victims of the disease and their fight for survival. She desperately wanted to be helpful. "I didn't want to be a doctor, so I had to look for other ways to be useful," she said. She became actively involved with many AIDS-related organizations and took classes that would help her make good arguments, so that she could debate healthcare issues. She used her strong intellect to compensate for feeling hopeless in the face of the suffering and deaths of her peers. Taking classes, she realized, would help her understand the latest research and would allow her to challenge policies and practices that were affecting her friends. Her mastery over her feelings of uselessness and hopelessness in the face of suffering sprang from her ability to debate issues and fight for change. Today Rachel continues to serve as an intellectual agent of change by drawing attention to issues of social and political injustice.

Even in her college years, Rachel's logic and passion can be seen—as in her senior thesis, "Identifiable Lives: AIDS and the Response to Dehumanization." In this thesis, she argues that an activist can exert influence by challenging the dehumanization of the gay population through rehumanization strategies. In essence, the argument was to make the unseen seen, by converting gay people into people with faces and stories, not just numbers. Her work was recognized by the Elie Wiesel Foundation in New York, winning the Elie Wiesel Prize in Ethics, which was created to foster civic responsibility and leadership in new graduates. Rachel's professor, John Cogan, described her as "one of the dozen best students I have taught at Stanford. I have never met any student who has her level of commitment and dedication to public service, bar none." Rachel graduated from Stanford early, having earned a degree in Public Policy with a concentration in Healthcare. She then went to work for the AIDS Coalition to Unleash Power (ACT UP), realizing that sometimes change can come only when active and militant steps are taken.

ACT UP is an international, non-partisan group that was started in 1987 to fight the AIDS crisis by bringing about changes in policy, medical research, and legislation. "I wasn't looking for a cause—I knew where I was and where I came from," Rachel said. She simply wanted to use her skills to make a social contribution—her way. She admitted that even though ACT UP was involved in many campaigns, protests, and group activities, she often went it alone. "I am not a joiner. I would go to meetings and be supportive, but then I would go and move into action and do my thing." She laughed. "I don't work well with others. I am often more productive and driven when I work alone."

The making of an activist seems to stem from an emotional or personal connection to an issue, and a willingness to do something even if it is a small first step. It entails the willingness to use our strengths and put them into action—not simply into conversation. When Rachel won a Rhodes Scholarship and traveled to England to work on her doctoral degree, she studied prison reform and AIDS. "There were people dying behind bars instead of in secure hospice facilities. It made no sense economically and was cruel," she explained. During her work with the ACLU on the National Prison Project, she advocated a reform of the existing policies of segregation of prisoners with HIV. Like others who identify themselves with a marginalized group, Rachel saw what many refused to see—social injustice. She was not indifferent but rather emotionally connected and moved to make a difference in the best way she knew: by making an intellectual argument and changing policy.

Become Intimate with Your Strengths

Historically, it seems to be in our nature to begin introspection with an analysis of our weaknesses, our obstacles, and our shortcomings. Until recently, the field of psychology focused on illness, deficits, and pathology almost to the exclusion of strengths and virtues. In the business world, strong leaders typically have been recognized for their ability to see what is not working at the systemic level and recognizing who is not capable at the personal level. Fortunately, we are now seeing a major shift in research, practice, and training toward the identification of strengths and the use of them to improve the bottom line, both in business and in the emotional well-being of individuals.

Identifying our life themes and the strengths that we possess is the foundation of success. Warren Buffet, one of the richest men in the world, once described his key to success as his ability to know his strengths and then make them better. He described himself as patient and practical—skills he uses every day in investing and running his business. Successful people, particularly women, learn to organize their lives in such a way as to maximize their strengths. And the discovery of our greatest strengths usually occurs under high-stress situations, when we default to what we can do best.

"Play full out," Susan Juris, CEO of a major hospital, would say at the conclusion of every leadership meeting. The phrase describes an energized state of mind that focuses on effort and action, allowing you to figure out what you need and then push through irrelevant and distracting tasks to meet that need purposefully. Those who "play full out" are not distracted by defeat or embarrassment and leave none of their skills unused; they demonstrate success in active motion. This was Susan's strength, and I had the opportunity to observe it during a time of crisis.

I first met Susan when I started to do some consulting work for the hospital where she worked. As a member of the senior leadership group, I had the privilege of learning and observing how Susan led her team—a diverse group of clinicians, administrators, and financial advisors, all with distinct ideas and experiences, which often led to spirited conversations.

In the fall of my second year of working with the hospital, there was an outbreak of Acinetobacter infection in our Intensive Acute Care area. The infection, resistant to many antibiotics and easily spread, increased the risk of medical complications and death among our most vulnerable patients. Tension increased as the facility went into high alert. Experts were consulted to offer guidance on room-disinfecting procedures, infection protocols, and strategies for containment. But, despite all efforts, the infection continued to spread. Patients were dying, fear was rising, and staff members were blaming each other for errors that contributed to the spread. Our smartest physicians managed their anxiety by doing what they did best—research. They set up conference calls and meetings with other clinicians across the country, looking for strategies of containment. Nursing staff set up stringent hand-washing and glove-changing procedures. Still with each day new cases appeared, and anxiety was very high.

During our many leadership meetings, I watched Susan as she listened to the experts, conducted a thorough analysis of the situation, and then used what I came to realize was her best strength—action. She first investigated innovative ideas that she had found in a local company piloting a novel technique to sterilize rooms. The next day she brought them, called town-hall meetings with the staff to reinforce protocols, and showed up on evening shifts to ensure that the strict hand-washing protocols were followed. She played to her strengths of action and a desire to learn and make connections from novel ideas.

I often wondered in the weeks that followed what would have happened if we had had a different CEO or if Susan's strength had lain in an ability to be deliberate and careful rather than prone to action. Perhaps the containment of the infection would still have occurred. But what I learned was the value of knowing and using your best strengths to achieve and thrive. That is how successful women step over their weaknesses and insecurities and actively master their strengths—they play full out.

Martin Seligman, in his book *Authentic Happiness*, points out that the greatest success and emotional contentment come from identifying and using our strengths rather than working on improving our weaknesses. Integrity, perseverance, social intelligence, courage, kindness, and leadership can all be improved with use and intention, and they tend to inspire others.

Since I am from Cleveland, Ohio, I have had the thrill of watching LeBron James play basketball. His innate athleticism is exciting and entertaining, but it does not inspire me to put on my tennis shoes and work on shooting hoops. On the other hand, watching him use his strength of generosity to help local children's organizations does inspire me. Talents themselves rarely inspire because most of us can't emulate natural talents that we don't possess. Strengths, on the other hand, can be nurtured and cultivated and, when observed by others, can inspire action.

Around the holidays, at the Starbucks coffee shop that I frequent far too often, it has become a common practice for strangers to pay for each other's orders. The first time this happened to me, I was so shocked that I didn't know how to respond. I remember pulling up to the window to pay for my order and being told that it had already been paid by the car that was now pulling away. There was no opportunity for me to thank the person, and clearly he or she was not asking for anything in return. The feeling that I was left with lingered as I drove to work, and I found myself not only smiling and singing but driving in a more courteous manner—slowing down to let cars cut in and avoiding the use of my horn. The cascading effect of a stranger buying me a Venti Chai Tea Latte that day changed my mood, my behavior, and my current Starbucks buying practice. I now make a conscious effort—not only during the holidays—to pay for the car behind me each time I go to the drive-through window.

The strengths of generosity and compassion are contagious and inspiring. When we use our strengths, we become our best, most authentic selves, and that yields happiness and success.

Failure: Where Success Begins

Another key ingredient for success is failure. Failing teaches us things that success simply cannot. The process of failing creates an internal alarm system that consciously and subconsciously guides our thinking and behavior as we learn new strategies. My grandmother, at 103 years old, continues to remind me that failing is the energy we need to fuel success. She says, "It is our failures that give us passion to push harder toward our purpose on earth." Failing shines a light on those strengths we have perhaps overlooked.

A balance needs to be struck between accepting failure and fearing it. Living in fear of failing can immobilize us and make us pass up opportunities for success and happiness. But the fear of failing, or atychiphobia, can also be a powerful motivator. It motivates Rachel, for example, to work harder, smarter, and better. She knows that she has landed her dream job—or, as she puts it, "won the job lottery." But getting there didn't happen because somebody made a phone call and opened a door for her. She got there on her own, persuading others that she could do the work. "Nobody put me here, so there is nobody to blame. I made the case that I can do this work, and if I fail that is a humiliation that I can't live with," she said.

While fear may be a motivator, success often acts as the stepping stone to more success. "Success is the best success," Rachel said. Although she acknowledged that people who are visible and "famous" are often considered role models for how to become successful, she shied away from framing what she means to others. "If my existence opens doors for others, then that is success." She laughed and added, "You know, a victory for women who wear sleeves on TV."

Rachel, like most of us, experienced many failures in her life journey, as she learned what she was good at and where she simply did not have skills. She knew from a young age that she was not the nurturing, hands-on, caregiving type. The idea of working in healthcare and standing by people's bedsides made her shudder. "I am not cut out for that kind of work," she said. But her gift of compassion and her intense belief in justice and the fair distribution of healthcare drove her to fight for those rights. She played to her strengths of compassion and intellect and thus helped to provide healthcare through a different window. Failing helps us dig in and discover what are and are not our gifts. Failing sets the stage for the active mastery of obstacles through the use of our unique strengths, and in this way it can act as the bridge to success.

That being said, actively mastering our fears and obstacles is not a one-and-done experience. It is a lifelong, conscious choice. Some days the shoes of mastery and confidence slip right on, and other days you need a shoehorn and some grease to force them on.

The Process of Mastering Our Struggles

Mari Smith, dubbed the queen of Facebook, understands this concept at a deep level. During a delightfully candid interview, she shared with me her own journey of mastering her shyness and poor self-esteem to become one of the world's greatest social-media thought leaders. Imagine a shy, quiet, insecure, and fearful young girl mastering the art of being social—speaking on a stage to large audiences, socially engaging in conversations on webcams, and communicating via social-media platforms to a million followers. Her story is the perfect example of using courage and innovation to actively master the passive struggle of insecurity.

Today Mari is a strikingly beautiful, tall, blonde, Scottish-Canadian woman. Her light blue eyes, hearty accent, and warm smile made it easy to engage with her in a deeply personal conversation about a time when she wasn't so confident.

In a recent trip back to the very rural area of British Columbia where she grew up, Mari visited her childhood home. "Looking at the house, it was so hard to imagine how my parents managed, with five children, with no running water, in such a primitive home," she said. Then she looked down, struggling with the tears that were forming. "As I stared at the path to the house, I saw my shy and scared little self," she whispered. "I sometimes still hear that little girl inside me, and I need to encourage her."

The seeds of self-doubt and insecurity can often begin in childhood, a time when we lack the ability to fully process and cognitively interpret experiences. One defining moment that placed Mari on a path of insecurity occurred when her parents came home with a Native American baby with special needs. Mari vividly remembers her father joyfully announcing that this was her new baby sister. Mari began to cry as she remembered the scene from long ago, recalling the chubby, dark-skinned, dark-haired little girl sitting on the floor. "I remember thinking to myself—why did they have to go and get another little girl? What is wrong with me?" This experience set the stage for her recurrent feeling of never being enough, which would be reinforced with every fight that her parents had and ultimately solidified when they divorced.

The fighting in the house was constant, as Mari remembers it. "As a child, I had many ear infections and digestive problems—clearly I did not want to hear or process the fighting." Finally, when Mari was twelve, she and her four sisters boarded a greyhound bus with their father to begin their journey back to Scotland. Her parents had divorced, and her father retained custody of the girls.

As Mari shared this story with me, she stared into the middle distance as if she were reliving that moment. "The bus was very crowded and loud, with few seats together. My little sister, who was only three, was crying." Her voice cracked as she added, "I looked out the window and saw my mother getting into her car, and I remember telling myself that I would never see her again. I convinced myself that the only way I could survive the pain was to think of her as dead—and that is what I did for ten years."

Stepping into Social Connections

Eventually Mari not only stepped into her big-girl shoes of courage and confidence, she designed them, manufactured them, modeled them, and sold them to others, becoming a world leader in social connections. Her path of connections began at the age of sixteen, when she completed high school and ventured into the workforce. "I had no interest in college. I couldn't wait to get out of school and begin to make my own money and be independent," she said. She remembered feeling eager to prove to her parents and herself that she could be successful in business and in relationships, so she set out on a journey to "show them how it could be done."

Using her curiosity, which she identified as her best strength, she began to teach herself everything from how to look good, feel good, and spiritually connect to how to speak in public, write a business plan, set up a website, and decorate cakes. She learned from books, correspondence courses, magazines, classes, and eventually the internet.

Although Mari held a variety of jobs in those early years, it was her cake-decorating skills that ultimately changed the course of her life. In 1998, she made the bold decision to start her own business. She spent a year preparing, with the plan to launch in 1999. "Then the universe dropped an invitation to come to San Diego," she said. With two suitcases and very little money, she arrived in the United States on a thirty-day return ticket. She knocked on doors looking for work and found herself doing many odd jobs. With time running out, literally on the twenty-ninth day of thirty, a call came from a local bakery that was looking for help with decorating Valentine's Day cookies and cakes. Standing tall in her big-girl shoes, with her portfolio of cakes tucked under her arm, Mari landed the job that would allow her to remain in San Diego and pursue her entrepreneurial dream.

She created a path for success one opportunity at a time: offering to speak at events, teaching small businesses how to build websites, and then teaching herself and others how to use social media to market their businesses. She took her curiosity and coupled it with hard work to create a thriving, international social-media consultancy and training agency and then to become a successful author and sought-after keynote speaker. Forbes named her as one of the top media power influencers, and she has been hired by Facebook to teach marketing to small businesses.

Despite these achievements, Mari's journey, like those of many other women, has been filled with failures, disappointments, and personal sacrifices. As her professional success grew, her marriage of eight years was ending. "I stayed about five years too long," she said with a sigh. "I realize now that I was motivated by trying to avoid the perceived pain of what my inner twelve-year-old self felt when my parent divorced. After all, I was determined to show my parents how a marriage could last. I would do it right. I got married later in life, mindfully chose a partner, and worked hard in therapy to make it last." But in the end Mari came to realize that ending the marriage was not a sign of failure but rather a choice—"a true choice for freedom."

The end of Mari's marriage left her with an easier last name, several years of pleasant memories, and an opportunity not only to stand in her big-girl shoes but to take a courageous step forward. Her business realized a record $500,000 in one week, and, best of all, for the first time she was able to stand in her mother's shoes and feel compassion for her.

When we actively master our hidden struggles, we become free to realize our greatest powers and to shine our light of courage and strength. This concept is not lost on Mari, who frequently whispers these beautiful words from Marianne Williamson: "Our deepest fear is not that we are inadequate. Our deepest fear is that we are powerful beyond measure. It is our light, not our darkness, that most frightens us."

CHAPTER 3

From Margin to Center: The Outsider
Fears Becoming an Insider

"When given the choice between fame and glory, take
glory. Glory has a way of sneaking up on fame and steal-
ing its lunch money later anyway."

— RACHEL MADDOW

MARGINALIZATION AS A social phenomenon is the process of moving certain
individuals or groups to the sidelines of society, where they are often
ignored and devalued. Their needs, views, experiences, and beliefs are
frequently seen as less important or valid than those of individuals in the
central and privileged positions of society. Religion, gender, age, sexual
orientation, homelessness, race, and financial status are just a few of the
criteria used in marginalization.

A strong commitment to social change and moral courage often
arise in those who have lived in the margins of life. Arguably, those
who have always resided in the privileged and popular center are too
distracted and distant to pay attention to scenes of injustice and prejudice. The sense of one's place in the world, of social responsibility,
and of connection to others seems the strongest in those who live
with oppression and are the recipients of prejudice and bias. It is for
this reason that many activists have expressed a fear that moving into
a privileged category may influence or change their compassion, their
empathy, and even their humanity. Yet several women who have been

marginalized for their race, culture, religion, sexual orientation, or gender have shared with me that they feel a need to recognize both their marginality and their privilege.

Privilege and marginality are not always mutually exclusive: a black woman may be the recipient of racial prejudice but experience privilege through being raised in a middle-class family; a Hispanic and homeless mother knows the oppression and stereotypes associated with both of these marginalized groups but may feel privileged because she is heterosexual and able-bodied; an affluent Jewish woman enjoys the privilege of a high social status but may experience prejudice directed at her Jewish heritage; and a poor white woman may feel privileged because of her race but oppressed because of her poverty.

Learning to examine our privilege does not erase or diminish the prejudice we experience or the pain of being marginalized; instead, it makes us mindful that it is possible to dance in both places. Being aware and mindful gives us the power to choose our actions and reactions. According to Margot Stern Strom, an international educator, leader, and social-change agent, smart and sensitive social and moral choices can best be made by combining education and self-examination.

"People Make Choices, and Choices Make History."

Margot Stern Strom has been described as a woman of compassion with a strong dedication to teaching through moral connection. Prior to interviewing Margot on these issues, I researched her personal and professional history. One of the first things I came across was an article in Harvard's *Ed. Magazine* entitled "Facing History, Facing Herself," by Lory Hough. Coincidentally, at the top of the article was a caricature of a woman, Margot, slipping big-girl shoes onto the tiny feet of two children—a symbolic gesture calling to mind rites of passage, teaching, and giving children the tools to approach painful historical issues and find the moral courage to walk. The article focused on Margot's retirement after four decades as the President and CEO of an organization that she founded back in 1976, called Facing History and Ourselves.

Margot began her professional career as a teacher of social studies at the Runkle School in Brookline, Massachusetts. She also studied moral development at the Harvard Graduate School of Education. During her teaching and training journey, it became clear to her that, in traditional teaching materials, the painful and difficult topics of history were at best summarized and at worst ignored. After attending a conference about the Holocaust, she realized that despite her Jewish heritage, her advanced degrees, and her years of teaching, she knew very little about that time in our history. It simply was not taught in any meaningful way. But not teaching about the Holocaust, racism, anti-Semitism, and violence in a morally challenging way seemed to her a denial of our responsibilities as human beings and democratic citizens.

With that realization, she set out on a journey to create learning materials that would challenge students and teachers to examine history through the filter of their own moral thinking—not simply provide factual historical information. Facing History and Ourselves (FHAO) was thus created. This once-small enterprise, which started with one innovative course, has now become a global organization. The teaching programs are used by more than 1.4 million high-school children around the world, in such countries as the United States, Switzerland, South Africa, Norway, the Czech Republic, and Peru, to name just a few.

As an international leader in education, Margot remains committed to challenging students to deal with the uncomfortable aspects of history, in an attempt to show them that we possess the power to do harm as well as good. The organization that Margot founded and ran for more than four decades continues to receive countless testimonials, including one from President Obama and First Lady Michelle Obama, who said, "[FHAO] is a great model. … It helps us use lessons from our history to guide compassionate informed decisions for the future." Actor Matt Damon was in the eighth grade when he was first exposed to and inspired by the program. He said, "It was the first time that history stopped being antiseptic to me. The lesson made it human—it was personal, and I was connected to it." He went on to say that meeting a woman who was a survivor of the Holocaust and hearing her story was one of the most deeply affecting things that had ever happened to him. Another student who completed the program said, "It is not His-story, it is Our-story." FHAO actively examines the intersection of historical facts and moral decision-making, which is one of the reasons that Steven Spielberg, award-winning director, producer, and film-writer, turned to FHAO when he wanted to tell the story of the Holocaust. His movie "Schindler's List" tells the story of Oskar Schindler, who saved the lives of more than 1,200 Jews during the Holocaust. Spielberg said, "Facing History came to my rescue when I wanted to tell the real story of the Holocaust and share it with students."

Margot focuses on the tag-line of the organization: "People make choices. Choices make history." Education for her is the marriage of ethics and knowledge, and it lies at the core of how we inform our choices. She has thought extensively about what was missing in the education of the German scientists and engineers who held PhDs and used their knowledge to build gas chambers for the concentration camps. She has come to the conclusion that what was missing was ethics—a moral dialogue mixed into the knowledge.

Margot has spent her professional life working to correct and enhance educational practices in order to create students who are "moral philosophers." Her international organization has succeeded beyond her wildest expectations. But how did Margot, a middle-school teacher, step into her own big-girl shoes and create this international movement? How did she use her marginality and privilege to influence how history is taught and examined all over the globe? That's where our conversation began.

Margot settled herself on her sofa as the sun shone through the window. She remarked what a lovely treat the morning had been: she had enjoyed her breakfast in a leisurely fashion. Retirement—it was a good thing! Just a month prior, after forty years, Margot had transitioned from her role as President of FHAO to President Emerita and Senior Scholar. But it took only a few minutes of the interview for me to realize that just because Margot was relaxing did not mean that this intellectually energetic woman would kick back and eat bonbons. On the contrary, she continues to create educational programs and experiences. Learning, teaching, and grappling with messy and painful moral issues are all in her blood. In fact, she waved one hand toward the books on her shelves as we spoke. "I am in regular dialogue with Eleanor Roosevelt, Lillian Smith, and other great figures in our history," she said. "I learn much about myself when I am talking to them."

At the beginning of our conversation, I shared a little about my grandmother, who had started me on a journey of learning about gratitude and aging. I told Margot about how Nana and I had written a book together that focused on her philosophy of life: in order to keep your passion and your purpose in full view, you must remain "greedy for life," maintaining an active pursuit of life by seeing more, learning more, and giving more; you must nurture both a greed for all that life offers and gratitude for that gift. Margot gently laughed and suggested that my grandmother was like a "living book on my bookshelf."

After I had explained the framework for our conversation and expressed my desire to learn more about her confidence and courage, Margot asked me to wait a minute while she got a pad and paper. She told me that often before an interview or a deep conversation, she makes a conscious decision as to whether or not she will do this. Today, she said, "I choose to have a pad of paper beside me as I am curious what I may say. I think this conversation about big-girl shoes and courage will be a lesson of discovery for me."

Written and Unwritten Rules of Hate

Margot started life with a curiosity and a desire to learn that were fostered by her parents. Her ideas and beliefs were shaped by the many books that filled the shelves in their family den. But, growing up in Memphis in the Jim Crow era, she learned even more from what wasn't taught. As a child, sitting in her classroom, she could see the Memphis Zoo across the street. Near the entrance of the Zoo a sign was clearly visible: "Colored day only on Thursday." It was just one of the many rules that people learned to follow but didn't discuss, living in the South in the 1950s. There were colored drinking fountains, colored waiting rooms, and a colored section on the bus. The segregation was visible everywhere, but it "never entered the classroom," Margot said. "We never discussed it, studied it, or acknowledged it."

In Lillian Smith's book *Killer of a Dream*, there is a chapter entitled "Customs and Conscience" that resonates with Margot. Lillian Smith, like Margot, grew up as a white child in the South when segregation was still in place. She writes, "I learned it was possible to pray at night and ride in a Jim Crow car the next morning and to feel comfortable doing both. I learned to believe in freedom and to glow when the word democracy was used and to practice slavery from morning until night. I learned it the way all my southern people learned it, by closing door after door until one's mind and heart and conscience are blocked off from each other and from reality."

Growing up in the segregated South had a lasting impact on Margot and her family. Her parents owned a furniture store in a predominantly black neighborhood, where they had many friends and customers who were black. They were visible supporters of Martin Luther King Jr., but the support came at a cost for the family. Margot has vivid memories of looking in their mailbox and finding hate letters and death threats to her brother, Gerald Stern. As a young attorney for the Justice Department's Civil Rights Division, Gerald was hated for his support of blacks. On the day that Martin Luther King Jr. was shot, riots erupted and the family furniture store was vandalized because of the signs in their window supporting the Civil Rights Movement.

Margot's brother, Gerald, was later quoted in *The Washington Post* as saying, "Though I was white, I identified with the blacks, with the victims, rather than with the White Southern establishment, so it was easy for me to imagine that their struggle was one I should join. I was able to imagine myself in the shoes of those black people, powerless, ignored;

maybe because that is the way I personally felt growing up in the South." Margot told me that, as a Jewish family living in the South, they were in fact marginalized in many ways. But Margot believes that their marginality gave them strength and a unique perspective from which to develop moral courage. Her family collectively used their gifts of intellect and social conscience to support and lobby for the rights of others.

Nevertheless, being seen as privileged or in the center of influence makes Margot uncomfortable. Reflecting on her brother, she said, "I just thanked him the other day for putting us on the right side of history. I am so proud of him and of my baby sister, Paula." The Honorable Paula Stern, PhD, served as the Chairwoman of the International Trade Commission in the Reagan administration and has been named as one of the top women influencing the American economy. "Paula and I share the same sensibilities, passion for justice, and shoes," Margot said, laughing. All three of the Stern children's lives were impacted by the Civil Rights Movement. Their parents established an environment in the home that focused on learning, justice, and the realization that change takes courage and often carries a price. Margot added, "The petri dish that was our family gave us permission for tolerance… Our marginality, as Jews in the South, gave us leniency to being human." Then she started to cry. "I watched those young black girls walk to the back of the bus—the shame they must have felt. I felt it too."

We Don't Belong on Pedestals

We can search for answers to why there is violence and hate by examining policies, laws, guns, mental illness, parents, teachers, and cultures, but the search will always lead us back to ourselves. In the end, our internal reflections are where responsibility and real change begins. In examining ourselves, we discover how easily we devalue others and ourselves in the process. As Margot reflected on her worth as a woman and her feelings of being an imposter, she got choked up. "I think women hurt each other when we put each other on pedestals. We devalue ourselves when we compare ourselves to a false image of successful women." She then shared a story that highlighted this battle.

While sitting in the waiting room of her dentist's office, Margot began a conversation with a man who was also waiting. He asked her what she did for a living, and she paused for a moment, knowing that explaining her organization and activities was not easy. When she began to explain about Facing History, the man's eyes grew wide, and he interrupted her, saying, "Oh, I know all about you. My wife loves you! You are her hero." As soon as he began to praise her, Margot shifted uncomfortably. She wondered where all of the praise was coming from, since she didn't even know his wife. It seemed strange that for all those years his wife had been putting her on a pedestal and seeing her only through the lens of her success with the organization. The man told her that his wife used to be a teacher and would be thrilled to know that he had run into Margot at the dentist. Margot asked for his wife's name and phone number. After her appointment, when she got into her car, she called her.

The woman answered the phone and was stunned to hear Margot's voice. She started to cry, "Oh, my God, I can't believe you are calling me!" Recollecting this woman's reaction as she spoke to me, Margot's voice cracked. She told me that she invited the woman to lunch so that they could have a conversation. Throughout the lunch, the woman continued to run herself down. She explained to Margot that she had once been a teacher but had then left the workforce to raise her children. She tried to explain what Margot represented to her. Margot was moved to tears as she remembered being viewed as a privileged and successful insider by this woman, while the woman demeaned her own choices.

At the end of the story Margot paused, thinking about the shoe metaphor. "I could not pull off those shoes that she thought I was wearing fast enough," she said. Margot understood the danger of being seen in only one way. That woman sitting across from her in the restaurant was struggling with her own worth. "She made many assumptions that I didn't struggle at times with *my* worth." The woman could not see the shared struggles between the successful woman sitting in front of her and herself, but the truth was that they had both made choices. Over the years, Margot had often chosen to give a talk, then hop on a plane home to be with her children instead of staying to network as many of her male colleagues did. She had brought her sick children to her office and frequently canceled important trips to be at home for school events.

"It was important to me that I didn't leave that restaurant with her still thinking that I was something I was not—and then by default thinking something less about herself," Margot told me. The story of this woman was a cautionary tale of how we as women often put each other on pedestals, framing each other one-dimensionally, and then by comparison diminish ourselves.

Margot's story reminded me that it is our natural, albeit unhealthy desire to place people into categories. Once people are in categories, assumptions and conclusions are more easily drawn. Margot told me that a woman once approached her after a talk she had given on genocide and said, "I didn't know you were Armenian." Her assumption was that only Armenians know and talk about genocide—just as sometimes people assume that only African Americans are interested in racism. How easy the black-and-white, concrete thinkers of the world have it. They never have to venture into the gray, murky waters where truth and injustice live.

Margot is inspired by people who recognize that stumbling is a way of going and not a failure in itself. "I think I learned this important lesson growing up marginalized. It allowed me to see the world through a different lens—like a microscope that you carry around, allowing you to see the deep and often dark issues."

Facing the Fear of Fame

The forecast had called for only an inch of snow, but over twelve inches had fallen already, and it was still snowing in Rachel Maddow's western Massachusetts home. Her red Ford pickup was buried under the snow. She began to shovel the driveway as the bitterly cold wind burned her face. Hours passed before she could even make her way to the truck.

Despite the frigid temperatures, she was sweating and peeled off layers of clothes as she worked.

Her thoughts were drifting back to her show. She climbed into the bed of the truck and began to shovel the heavy snow from the top of the cab. In that moment, she thought about how different her current reality was from the one she had left just twelve hours earlier. The amount of ego it takes to work in media had been making her worry about how it might be changing her. Would she even like herself when all of it ended? Images flashed through her mind.

She thought back to 11:00 am on a Monday morning, when she put on her tennis shoes and began her jog to the studio. Running was a new-found exercise for her. Her winter hat was on, her glasses perched on her nose, and her scarf was wrapped tightly around her neck. Most people who passed her on the street probably didn't recognize her, and those who did were usually fans with kind words.

As she approached the entrance to 30 Rockefeller Center, her mind moved to the work at hand. Topics, news stories, guests, and the preparations that needed to be completed before she went live at 9:00 pm. With her mind preoccupied, she entered the office area. A new, entry-level staff-member recognized her and backed up to the wall as she passed him. It bothered her. When had she become that person? It was a disturbing thought that came back during her staff meeting.

Her staff meetings typically begin at 2:00 pm. By that time, she has typically already been working in her office for five hours. She has read seven newspapers and catalogued a list of potential topics to use for the show. The daily meetings are held in the center of her staff's cubicle space, where Rachel stands before a whiteboard and everyone brainstorms ideas for the seven segments of the show. Some topics are readily dismissed, while others are challenged to the smallest detail. Standing with her back to the staff as she writes on the board with her usual laser-focused concentration, acutely aware of their time constraints, Rachel can sense the tension in the air. "The room tends to get silent as I am writing—I can get real intense," she said. I myself had observed that intensity first-hand, the night before my interview with her, as I watched her during her live broadcast in studio.

She grimaced as she explained to me that in addition to her own staff, staff from other shows often arrive to observe the process. "There is such an intensity around these meetings," she said. Ideas are shared, strategies discussed, and guests booked before the live show in the evening. Rachel is very much aware of her level of intensity and the fact that her staff can become intimidated—holding back and hesitating to raise their hands.

She is acutely sensitive to the nagging silence in the room. "I feel like the Wizard of Oz," she confided in me, saying that she feels bothered by the ongoing fear that this kind of power can become, as she put it, "toxic to the soul." She worries about her identity being lost in her work; she is afraid that she may not like who she has become when the job ends. "It actually keeps me up at night," she added. Because of these fears, she tries to remain vigilant about not losing her real self to her fame.

When she first started in the media industry, many people advised her to adopt the "no new friend" policy. She was warned that she would meet people who wanted to be her friend solely because of her position of power. The rebellious side of Rachel did not believe this would apply to her, and she tried to prove it wrong. Unfortunately, the advice turned out to be quite sound—as she learned the hard way. She now admits to keeping the "no new friend" policy in place. However, she worries that this will lead to a limited existence, as she holds on only to friends from her pre-fame era and develops social relationships only with other people in her industry, leading to a more homogeneous group than she is comfortable embracing. In the end, though, she is mindful of the risk of being taking advantage of and the need to remain selective about whom she accepts as friends. For now, the "no new friend" rule is being enforced.

With a smile, I suggested that present company should be excluded. She laughed.

Dancing in the Margin and the Center

Living as part of a marginalized group is fraught with struggles and pain—consequences that are not typically seen as desirable. However, some people argue that living in the margins has given them the gifts of tolerance, resilience, courage, and leniency toward others. The marginalized "other" is often invisible, with no voice, no representation, no advocates, no rights, and no power—or so it seems. But on closer examination, those who are not seen are often those who see, feel, and react to injustice with a powerful force.

Marginalized "others" often fear losing their true selves and becoming part of the privileged establishment. Rachel Maddow battles with this fear as she worries about who she will be when her work ends. There seems to be a need in her for hypervigilance and self-checking, to be mindful of her authority and privilege in order to remain who she is at the core. Rachel's strategies are both internal and external.

The balance she consciously works to achieve is physically noticeable. In her television life, we as viewers see the top half of Rachel: a nondescript, rotating stock of gray, black, and navy suit jackets—the wardrobe of the job. But underneath the anchor desk is the real Rachel, who stands firmly in her signature tennis shoes and baggie 501 Levi jeans. These serve as reminders of her true self—a sort of ego-check strategy. In fact, when Rachel won the prestigious Rhodes Scholarship in 1995, she held true to her promise to dye her hair blue. It was a gesture that said, "I am still me, not one of them"—not one of the privileged establishment.

While writing her doctoral dissertation, Rachel did many interesting and odd jobs—including yardwork. Yes, the Rhodes Scholar, Emmy-Award-winning television host, AIDS activist, Stanford graduate Dr. Maddow can also rip out tree trunks. Moreover, she is a competent mixologist, barista, and coffee-bean bucket cleaner. But the thing she labels as her best accomplishment is her deeply committed relationship to her partner of seventeen years, Susan.

Rachel, scruffy and dirty, was working in Susan's yard doing landscaping work when Susan opened the door. Rachel fell in love immediately. She describes Susan as the "spine on which the rest of the bones of my life happen—it is miraculous." The most successful way that Rachel has discovered to keep herself real is her relationship with Susan. She splits her time between her apartment in New York and her home in western Massachusetts, where she returns every weekend. Going home is one of her best strategies in her battle not to become somebody she won't recognize or like when her fame ends. "Our home is in a rural area where most people don't even have cable, so they have no idea how I am doing in the ratings or care," she told me, laughing. There is nobody waiting to chauffeur her around or seek her out for their own agenda.

Rachel described going home as "getting on Susan's ride," saying that Susan "dials her back." Susan challenges Rachel when she feels that Rachel has brought home her work identity, attitude, or expectations. She is the balancing force for Rachel. "I run the errands, cut the wood, recycle, walk the dog, and get the groceries," Rachel said. Then she added with another laugh, "And if I get the wrong stuff—I am sent back to the store." She credits this normal life and routine with keeping her from becoming complacent about things like having a car waiting whenever she wants to go anywhere in New York, or the fact that nobody ever challenges her thoughts and ideas but only gives ingratiating compliments.

These seemingly disconnected images—a Stanford graduate, Rhodes Scholar, PhD, and wildly successful radio and television personality on the one hand, and a marginalized, radical, lesbian activist on the other—are held together within this complex woman. Rachel has found a style that allows her to remain "other," with all the leniency, tolerance, and compassion that comes from being marginalized, while also holding the privilege of being celebrated and famous. She has changed the image of what a popular, funny, smart, and successful woman can look like—dancing with one foot in the privileged center and the other in a marginalized group.

Confronting Blame from Others and the Self

Being marginalized can erase a person from the view of others—making them seemingly invisible, misunderstood, and judged. Betsy was one of those unseen young women. She was only eighteen years old when she first came to my office for therapy. She entered the room and positioned herself on the edge of the couch, with her head hanging low and her hands held tight together in her lap. Her long brown hair fell to the middle of her back, and her dark brown eyes were swollen and bloodshot from hours of crying. She wore black stretch pants and an oversized sweatshirt, but her six-month's-pregnant belly was still visible. As she gently eased back into the sofa, she put her face in her hands and began to sob.

Betsy came from an abusive home, with a controlling and angry mother who frequently told her daughter that she was worthless, had ruined her mother's life, and had driven her father to drink. Betsy was frequently called "a mistake." She learned to cope with the verbal abuse, but when the sexual abuse started and her mother made excuses, saying that her father was drunk and therefore wasn't responsible, she knew she had to leave. She stayed with friends just long enough to graduate from high school, and during that time she used drugs to numb herself and sex to feel connected to others. Now that she was pregnant, the friends she had been staying with didn't want her anymore.

When she first learned that she was pregnant, she went to an abortion clinic and sat in the parking lot. How could she take care of a baby when she couldn't take care of herself? She went back to the clinic several days in a row, trying to convince herself that it was the right decision. But in the end she decided to bring the baby to term and then maybe give it up for adoption. With nowhere else to go, she moved into a homeless shelter.

A colleague of mine who was volunteering at the shelter first introduced me to Betsy. The call came one evening: could I offer a few crisis appointments for Betsy to help her cope with her circumstances and the depression she was battling? Those few sessions turned into a few years of therapy. In her very first appointment, with tears running down her face, Betsy looked me in the eye and told me that she was not worthless. She reassured me that she was working at a local diner and would be able to make the payments for my services.

Remembering that moment still moves me to tears. I was witnessing raw courage, and I felt hugely inspired by Betsy's bravery in coming to my office, with her shame and fear clearly exposed, yet armed with the strength to fight for her dignity and the self she was trying to understand.

I saw Betsy for five years—through the birth of her son, her move from the shelter to a subsidized apartment, and her advancement from an entry-level job in the food industry to a management position at the same restaurant. I watched her network with other single mothers to share babysitting responsibilities, which allowed her to take evening classes at a community college. I watched her raise her son alone while she actively participated in therapy, working on parenting strategies and self-esteem.

Betsy was a marginalized mother. She was not a white, middle-class, married woman. She was a Hispanic, unmarried woman who lived homeless for a year. Being a homeless mother means being considered by almost everyone to be a "bad" mother. Other mothers believed that Betsy had gotten herself into the mess by getting pregnant and not working hard enough to make enough money to provide for her child. Sometimes she herself believed this view of her situation. It was a daily struggle to confront the devaluation by others and herself.

Thirteen years later, long after our last session, a package was delivered to my office. Inside was a picture of a young man wearing a high-school cap and gown and a beaming woman with her arms around him. The note attached read simply, "Thank you for seeing me and for making me see myself. Gratefully, Betsy." Her marginalization forced her to cultivate her own beliefs, to build support structures with other mothers who were in similar situations, and to resist the expectations and rules set by mothers at the privileged center of society. Betsy found her strength in being part of the "other"—the homeless mother who was also a good mother—and so she moved from the margins to the center of society: her own center as she defined it.

Transforming Adversity to Honor

William Barclay, a Scottish author and minister, once said, "Endurance is not just the ability to bear a hard thing, but to turn it into glory." Betsy endured her hardships and transformed the image of a homeless mother both for herself and for others. Her life and example of courage won her the praise and honor of her community. Betsy was not famous, but in the end she was someone. She was a private hero for herself, her son, and the other women who saw in her the possibility of a life of dignity and value.

Rachel Maddow, in her commencement address to the 2010 class of Smith College, implored the graduates to learn the difference between fame and glory, to see personal triumphs as overrated if they don't lead to the greater good of others. "When given the choice between fame and glory, take glory," she said. "Life might very well be long. Keep your eyes on the horizon and live in a way that you will be proud of. You will sleep more, you will be a better partner, you will be a better mom, you will be a better friend, and you will not have to remember any complicated lies to brag about at the old-age home, because you can brag about the truth of your well-lived life."

PART II

When the Other Shoe Drops: Fostering Resilience

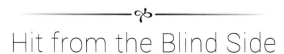

CHAPTER 4

Hit from the Blind Side

"Ever notice that the things we worry about most in life
are usually the things that never happen?"

— Stefani Schaefer, Emmy-Award-winning Fox 8 news
anchor, Cleveland, Ohio

The phrase "waiting for the other shoe to drop" comes from the manufacturing boom of the late nineteenth and early twentieth centuries, when crowded tenement living in New York City exposed neighbors to each other's intimate sounds. It was not uncommon for neighbors to hear each other taking off their shoes. But it wasn't so much the sound of the first shoe hitting the floor that caused annoyance as the anticipation of waiting for the inevitable second one to hit the floor.

Today this idiom means to wait for something that is unavoidable because it is linked to a previous event. The connotation is that it is not only unavoidable but negative. You never hear people "waiting for the other shoe to drop" in connection with something good. Instead, the phrase implies that something bad is coming—and that it is not a matter of if but when. Psychologically, waiting of this kind creates anticipatory anxiety. We wait, we anticipate, we remain vigilant and anxious that more negative events will follow, or else we engage in superstitious thinking, telling ourselves that if everything is going well in our lives we should brace ourselves because something bad is surely coming—the dreaded "other shoe."

The problem with this habit is that it makes us waste much of our lives worrying about what may be coming in the future. We keep our bodies and our minds in a heightened state of tense readiness. Some people even make a conscious effort to contain their joy and contentment so that, when the other shoe inevitably drops, they will be prepared and it won't hurt as much.

Worry, defined as a chain of thoughts and images usually associated with negative and at times uncontrollable emotions, can be either valuable or dangerous, depending on how we act upon it. Worrying about small, day-to-day things can serve to motivate us into action, for example by making a doctor's appointment or problem-solving around an identified crisis. But when we engage in chronic worry about things that are anticipated or hypothetical—the "what if" and "Oh my God" kind of thinking—it can be harmful to our emotional and physical health. It holds us in a state of heightened emotional arousal and thus activates our fight-or-flight response. As we wait and prepare to move into action, our blood pressure and heart rate remain elevated and adrenaline chronically circulates. But if the things we are worrying about never happen, our body never has the opportunity to react and expend the energy. We stay indefinitely in a state of "readiness," which can deplete the emotional resources that are critical for us to tap into when faced with actual emergencies—those moments we don't see coming, the ones that hit us from the blindside without warning.

In everyone's life there comes that blindside moment—a moment when we are slapped out of complacency, out of our mundane, structured routine, out of our daily complaints and worries, out of our perspective of the world and of ourselves. That moment when the life we created becomes a distant image in the rearview mirror, when we catch a glimpse of ourselves and are forced to confront our vulnerabilities and our resilience. That moment when we are brought to our knees and our emotional selves want to curl up and quit, but we are forced to stand up tall, put on our big-girl shoes, and dig deep to cultivate hope.

Stefani Schaefer, a popular news anchor in Cleveland, Ohio, knows first-hand what it is like to be hit from the blindside with tragedy.

When the Brain Reacts to Fear

I first met Stefani on the set of WJW Fox 8 in Cleveland, more than twenty years ago. As a psychological contributor for the local media, I was interviewed many times over the years by Stefani—or Sissy, as her friends call her. Professionally, I found her to be warm and engaging, and personally, as an interviewer, the same. Her infectious smile and genuine warmth made her easy to communicate with on any topic that we were discussing on air. Over many years, our paths continued to cross, both during her time at WJW Fox 8 and during her tenure at WEWS Channel 5 in Cleveland. A warm friendship developed, and the time we spent together was filled with a lot of laughter, a great emotional connection, and a shared love of chocolate.

Voted the most popular news anchor in the city, Sissy is beloved by many of her viewers and followed by more than 114,000 fans on Facebook. As the co-anchor of the WJW Fox 8 morning show, she is visible to us daily, and through social media and her presence in the community, Sissy has become even better known. Her fans celebrate her personal joys and champion her professional causes. We have enjoyed seeing photos over the years of her family: her husband, Roger, and children, Race and Siena. And we clung to the Facebook picture of her and her husband and children on the shores of Kauai, Hawaii, where, only four months before the tragedy, they celebrated their wedding anniversary.

That happy family image was floating in my own head when I reached for the phone and dialed Sissy. My hands were shaking, and I knew I would have no words but could offer only what others were offering—my prayers and loving thoughts. She picked up the phone on the first ring. We both started to cry.

The day that the other shoe dropped for Sissy was a rainy, cool, April day on the shores of Lake Erie. The familiar hustle of the morning routine began in Sissy's home. Race and Siena were getting ready for school while chatting about play practice. They were both in the school play, "Annie," and the first performance was just a few weeks away. Siena had the lead role of Annie, just as her mom had many years earlier.

Sissy yelled a few reminders down the stairs about items that the kids needed to take to school. She told them that she would pick them up after school and that they would head straight to practice. "I love you guys. Have a great day," she yelled as they departed. As usual, her husband, Roger, yelled things down to them as well, but his were silly comments that made them laugh. Roger, the jokester of the family, provided the humor. He called to Race, "Remember to say hi to Monday Mary and Tuesday Tom"—a private joke that made Race belly laugh. A final call came down to them: "I will meet you guys in the car." Roger then poked his head into the bathroom and had a quick, light discussion with his wife about their weekend plans. It was the playful and familiar banter that comes from fourteen years of marriage. He smiled, and then out the door he went. It was a typical Friday morning.

Sissy pushed open the sliding door to her closet and stepped in to select her outfit for the day. The anchors on the Fox 8 morning show all wear similar colored clothing, and today, she reminded herself, was purple day. She slipped into her purple short-sleeved blouse, her black skirt, and her gold-heeled, leopard-print, sling-back pumps. While clearly not the most comfortable shoes, they are a great look for television. Indeed, they are part of the big-girl uniform: professional, sophisticated, and stylish.

She arrived at the station and began to review the content and segments for the show. The cooking segment would involve grilling outside in the parking lot; the band was setting up for the second hour; guests were arriving and being sent into the green room. The show was fun and playful, and so was the tone in the studio.

As the show wrapped up and the cameras turned off, Sissy removed her microphone from the lapel of her blouse and placed it in the usual spot for the next crew. Her colleagues, Wayne and Kristi, said their goodbyes and left the building. Sissy stayed behind to give a tour of the station to an old high-school friend, and an hour later, around 11:00, she returned to her desk in the newsroom.

There on top of her desk sat a copy of the local paper, *The Plain Dealer*, and on the front page was a picture of Roger in his hard hat, standing on scaffolding as he put solar panels on the roof of a church. The photo had been taken the day prior for an article on the church renovation that Roger was leading. He worked in construction and was particularly proud of the work being done on the church. Sissy laughed as she saw the paper and told a co-worker that she was going to call him to tease him about his celebrity status. She reached for the phone but then decided that she would wait and call him privately from the car. Wrapping up a few details at her desk, she looked at her watch and grabbed her purse. Just then her phone rang. It was Roger's boss.

That moment. The moment when our brain hears and interprets words being said but our emotional and intuitive side has yet to react. She heard a voice saying, "Stef, there has been an accident. Roger fell off some scaffolding at work, and he is a little out of it. The ambulance has arrived and is taking him to the emergency room." Time stopped.

Under normal circumstances, the brain will allow information to float in and then out like a sieve—scanning for any novel or important information that requires attention. This is the reason that we can multi-task and zip through our mundane tasks: the brain is essentially on auto-pilot. However, when a crisis or trauma occurs, the brain becomes vigilant and time slows to allow us to process what is happening. There is no frame of reference or existing template in the brain to tell us how to respond to unique traumatic events. This is the reason that under emergency situations, time seems to stand still. It does so to help us process and react.

In that moment, Sissy felt as if everything had slowed to a crawl—time, movement, sounds, even her thoughts. She was trying to make sense of what she was hearing. Focus. What was he telling her? She replayed the words in her mind. Then her heart started to race as she heard something else in the call, something that wasn't being said. A blur—the details of the words were out of focus. She let out an involuntary yell, dropped the phone, and took off her beautiful, leopard-print, sling-back shoes. Her co-workers heard the scream and saw her running. Time felt distorted. She sprinted down the hallway, carrying her shoes. It was a hallway that she had walked down thousands of time over the years, but in that moment it seemed unusually long, and her legs felt heavy and slow.

Her thoughts were spinning as words and phrases began to run through her head: "he is out of it," "ambulance taking him," "call my mom," "what about the kids." Then her thoughts became focused. Run. Run fast. As she was telling me this story, much later, the memory made her eyes fill with tears. She reached for a tissue and took a deep breath. Her voice trailed off as she recalled the raw fear she had felt as she ran down the hallway of the news station, out to the parking lot, and into her car, still in her bare feet, carrying her shoes—her big-girl shoes that earlier that morning had made her feel pretty, confident, and capable. She didn't feel like that anymore. She felt scared, alone, and weak.

Fear: The Mind in Slow Motion

As she drove to the hospital, Sissy's mind was racing with thoughts, fears, and images. Anxiety was setting in, and she felt her bare foot on the accelerator getting numb and heavy. She forced her mind back to the task at hand. She reached for the phone and called Roger's sister, his mother, and then her own mother. It was during that last call, when she heard her mother's voice, that true panic took over and her tears started to flow.

The first call when bad things happen is usually to our mothers or the parental figures in our lives—we reach for their wisdom and guidance. We want to step out of our big-girl shoes and into the passive role of a child. Reaching out to a parent in times of crisis seems to be a universal response.

At this point in our talk, Sissy paused, tears in her eyes, and looked up at me. She said, "If the kids were injured or sick, the first call I would make would be to my mom. Under usual circumstances, she would listen and then tell me she was on her way. Then I would respond, 'No, you stay there. Let's wait and see if this is serious.'" This was the comfortable and common routine between them. But this time, when her mom offered to come, Sissy responded, "Good. Please hurry." As she hung up the phone, her foreboding about the horror that would soon be revealed settled into the core of her being. She felt nauseated and light-headed. Focus, she thought. Focus.

The drive to the hospital, pulling into the emergency-room entrance, and parking the car are foggy memories for Sissy even today. But she does vividly recall grabbing her sling-back shoes, putting them on, and rushing through the emergency-room doors. Once inside, she felt lost and confused. She began to wander through the hallway, the waiting area. Focus. Focus! She willed her brain to take in details so that she could figure out what was happening. Where is he? Who do I ask? Where do I go?

She recalls somebody recognizing her and escorting her to a small room. The woman, with the somber face, informed her that she had beaten the ambulance to the hospital and that they would let her know when it arrived. Time seemed to slow to a crawl again. The room felt cold, and its walls were stark. It contained only a few chairs and a table. On that table sat a box of Kleenex. Sissy looked at the box, and her nausea returned. She eased herself into a chair as she saw familiar faces being escorted into the room. Roger's family arrived, and her longtime friend and colleague, Wayne, joined her. She began to cry—or had she been crying since the call, since that life-changing moment?

There was no clock, but it didn't matter. Time was irrelevant as she waited to hear about what had happened to her husband. In the distance, the sound of sirens could be heard. Her heart was pounding. She reached for Wayne's hand as a doctor in scrubs appeared in the doorway. He came in and sat across from her. He took a deep breath and said, "Your husband has sustained a severe head injury, and we are going to life-flight him to Metro Hospital."

The words seemed so heavy. Sissy looked at Wayne and began to cry, blurting out, "You know what that means—they want him in that hospital so they can harvest his organs. They think he is brain-dead." Her mind flashed to numerous news stories that she had reported about organ harvesting at the trauma center. She began to sob and begged to see Roger before they put him in the helicopter. They agreed.

She stood, but her legs were weak and the high-heeled shoes offered little support. She wasn't confident, capable, or strong in that moment. Wayne put his arms around her and assisted her and Roger's mother into a small and crowded room. A clinical team of eight to ten people were hustling around, attending to intravenous poles, transport materials, charts, and other apparatus. Sissy's eyes went straight to Roger, who was lying on the gurney, covered in blood. She ran to his side, put her hands on his face, and cried out, "Don't leave me. Don't leave us! Fight. Fight! We are here. We need you. I love you." His body jerked in response. He would fight with everything he had. She knew that. She felt that. It was the last time that he would know her or respond to her—his wife.

The clinical team prepared Roger for the flight. As the helicopter took off, Sissy ran to the parking lot and got into the passenger seat of Wayne's car. While en route to Metro Hospital, Sissy started to pray, at first to herself and then out loud with Roger's mother, who was sitting in the back seat. Wayne was driving at record speed. She looked out the window and saw other cars, billboards, road signs—but nothing was registering. It was all just a haze, much like her thoughts. As she prayed and looked up at the sky, she noticed that the life-flight helicopter was following the same path to the hospital. She kept her eyes on it and yelled out, "Fight, Roger! Fight! I am here. Don't leave me."

The memory of that moment still causes Sissy to shake. As she told me about it she took a sip of water, her hands trembling. "I think it was the moment when the knot tightened hard in my stomach and a new foreboding feeling was stirring," she said. She recalls consciously pushing that feeling away by praying louder, drowning out her fearful thoughts.

Upon their arrival at the hospital, time seemed to stand still again, but at the same time the activity around her sped into fast forward. She was approached by the clinical team, who explained to her that quick decisions would need to be made. They told her about an experimental drug that was showing great promise for traumatic brain injury but had to be administered within the first few hours. It would be given as an IV drug for the next five days. The drug had been shown in several studies to improve survival rates. Did she want to use it on Roger? Her response was quick. "Yes. Yes, of course, give it to him and hurry. He is a fighter, and he would want us to do everything to help him fight. There is no decision to be made." She looked to Roger's mother, who nodded her head in agreement.

But the doctor paused long enough for her to see something dark reflected in his face. "What is the risk to this medication?" she asked.

"It sometimes saves the lives of those that God would otherwise take," he said. Sissy heard his words, but her brain filed them away to be processed later—much later. Right then, keeping him alive, giving him the best odds to fight and live, was her focus. The medication was administered, and the journey began.

Balancing Public and Private Grief

Because Sissy is a public figure, articles appeared in the newspaper regarding the injury, and her station issued a public statement. She knew she would not be leaving Roger's bedside and certainly would not be returning to work for a while. Calls and emails flooded in, food was sent, flowers arrived, and prayer circles formed. While the crisis that she and her family were now enduring was private in many ways, she also knew that support and prayers from friends and fans would comfort her. So, eight days after her darkest moment, she sat down to write a public statement on her Facebook page.

When she opened the page, she saw her last entry, which she had meant as a simple inspirational thought of the day. It read, "Ever notice that the things we worry about most in life are usually the things that never happen?" She had posted it on April 18th, 2012, just eight days before her life had changed forever. What an eerie foreshadowing, an ironic reminder that we expend so much of our emotional energy worrying about things that never happen—the big, the little, and the insignificant. It is as if we think that worrying will protect us or prepare us.

That evening Sissy reached out to her support network. She took a deep breath and shared her story with all who were supporting her and Roger:

May 5th, 2012, Facebook: Stefani Schaefer Fans

Dear friends. Last Friday, April 27, my world collapsed. My husband, best friend and soul mate fell 12 feet off scaffolding while working at a construction site. He was rushed to Hillcrest and once they realized his head trauma was so extensive and severe, he was life-flighted to a level 1 trauma center. I was able to see him just before he was life-flighted—Wayne carried me and Roger's mom into that room. It was the most horrific sight I had ever experienced—I held his face and told him how much I loved him, that he was my world, I told him to keep fighting, talked about Race and Siena. He was reacting—it was amazing. I know he heard every word I said. Roger was diagnosed with severe head fractures, severe brain bleeding and brain bruising. Friday evening, the swelling got to be too much, so doctors performed a craniotomy, where they removed the side of his skull to allow the brain to swell outside and not down to the brain stem which would be fatal. That night, my mother brought our children Race and Siena to the hospital—we were told for them to be there. During surgery, my children, mother, Roger's mom, my friends, many of my co-workers and even some of my bosses, picked me up off the floor, held me and prayed with me. We said the Rosary all during Roger's surgery. It made us all feel so strong during my darkness hours. That group of amazing people gave me strength to want to live—because I was dying inside. That surgery and all the prayers saved him that night—NO question. He is still in a coma and has been fighting for his life every single moment since then. His strength blows me away (and I think the doctors might be pretty impressed too). This past week has been such a blur for me, as I have been in such a state of shock, disbelief and complete and utter grief. But I have to keep going, for Roger and for our children. This week, I have experienced more ups and downs than I ever knew existed. The bad news comes like a blow to the stomach with a bat. The tiny good news makes me run into a little room and jump up and down like a little girl, get on my knees and praise God. I can't even begin to tell you how supportive my family at Fox 8 has been. They were there with me every step of the way. They hold prayer groups for Roger, they text me positive thoughts, they are even taking turns bringing us dinner every night. Their love blows me away. What a place and I have never felt more honored to be a part of that beautiful news station. So many people from all the other stations have reached out to me. It's amazing how in times like these, we all become one. My children's school has been incredible too... they have had prayer groups and are carrying Race and Siena through this. All of our friends have been incredible. My sweet friends are taking me to the hospital every day and even staying with us every night, because that's when it's so lonely. Roger is now not allowed visitors, calls, flowers, etc. because of his very critical state. But what I am begging from all of you... is prayers. My sweet friend Pastor Rob, The Nemehs, our priests at our parish, Sister Sheeley, Wayne Dawson, Bill Martin. The list goes on and on with the ministers/priests who have prayed over my baby. All of my friends, people we have never met are praying for Roger. And that is why I am able to be here at this moment, telling you, those prayers are WORKING! There is no doubt. I beg you, as my friends, to pray for my Roger. Please for a moment pray for that sweet man. I can't thank you enough. I don't know when I will return to work. Now all I can think about or focus on is Roger and our children. I do know that I want to work while he is in brain rehab—because once he is here with us, I want to spend as much time as I can with him. Thank you for your prayers! Stef

The days came and went. Race and Siena went to school and came home, but the house was changed. There was no regular dinnertime, and when they did eat together it was quiet. There were no jokes, no laughter, and

69

no Dad. There was only homework, play practice, school activities, and bedtime. Everybody went through the motions. After a few weeks, Sissy returned to work; she put on her big-girl shoes and did her job with grace and professionalism. But it was all changed. Now her phone was never out of her sight or reach. She would receive and send text messages during commercial breaks. When the number was unfamiliar, she answered the phone on the first ring and then held her breath. Her energy did not come easily or naturally. She was barely sleeping or eating and found it increasingly difficult to concentrate. She interacted with guests, her colleagues, and her children, but she was not fully present, mentally or emotionally. Conversations and interviews would be going on, but her thoughts would be running on a different track. She would be thinking about numbers—Roger's numbers.

Over the next several months, Roger underwent numerous surgeries; he suffered seizures, infections, and complications; and he moved in and out of consciousness. There was always a running calculation in Sissy's head: how many days have passed since the injury, since his last surgery, since his last seizure, since the start of his newest antibiotic? She knew that the number of days was important for his prognosis. Each day that passed affected the time it would take for him to improve and return home.

During one of her broadcasts, her thoughts bounced back to her most recent conversation with the physician about her husband's intracranial pressure, another number that would become part of her daily vocabulary. She learned that the intracranial pressure (ICP) is the pressure caused by an increase in fluid surrounding the brain. When it rose to 25mm Hg they had had to perform the craniotomy to relieve the pressure, and then, when it rose again to 20 mm Hg, Roger had had a seizure. Last night it had hovered at the upper limit of normal, 15mm Hg. Had it risen again? She made a mental note to text the nursing staff during the commercial break. She said a quiet prayer that it would not rise and then shifted the thought to the back of her mind as she welcomed the next guest to the show.

Sissy also moved through the everyday tasks involved in taking care of her young children. Her son, Race, was eleven, and Siena had just turned ten. Sissy went to work, cooked, plunged toilets, and so on, but without full conscious awareness. Trauma creates chaos in the brain. The nonverbal, emotional side of the brain takes over, while the intellectual, problem-solving frontal cortex sits idle. The brain numbs itself to reason and registers either the traumatic experience or nothing at all. This is the protective mechanism of shock. It keeps everything a bit out of focus, allowing the person to process slowly and cope with only small pieces at a time.

The front of Sissy's mind was filled with the mundane motions of living, while her every conscious thought focused on how to get Roger back. She was determined to make him better. In the midst of crisis, we often turn to what we know, our usual strategies for coping, and for Sissy this meant being in control. By her own admission, she is a Type A, high-energy person. She told herself that she needed to set a goal and make it happen. She recalled saying to her children, "We can do this. We can bring Daddy back. We will love him back. We will care for him and help him back. I can fix this. This is in our hands now—we are his family."

Control: we try to grab it with both hands when fear is present. A process unfolds in which we desperately manage every detail, trying to control every outcome and anticipating every step that needs to be taken. A frantic need for total control—and no mistakes—arises in us. The need to succeed is intense, as the stakes for failing are too high and too intolerable.

For the next six months, Sissy slept very little and ate even less. She began to look frail, thin, and exhausted. Her already slight figure lost twenty pounds, and her hair started to fall out. She found sleep only in brief periods in the chair next to Roger's hospital bed, or for a few hours at home. Her mind would not allow her to rest. She was on a mission, and she would not fail. Roger was going to get better and return home by Thanksgiving, then by Christmas, then by Valentine's day. But each holiday came and went. Roger was not able to return home.

Although Sissy occasionally caught a glimpse of herself in the mirror and thought, "I need to eat something," she had no desire for food and no energy to think about eating. She recalled during our talk that there were times when she would drag herself home from the hospital and begin to prepare her kids for bed—only to have them remind her that they had not even had dinner. She admitted that if it had not been for the kindness of her colleagues and friends, who brought meals in every day, the family might have had no meals at all. Eating wasn't her focus. Her mind was focused on making her husband well. While he was in a coma, she would sit and talk to him, praying over him and hoping he would respond, remember, return.

Over the months that followed, he started to show progress, and Sissy's spirits lifted. Though he was not yet communicating with her, hope was renewed. He woke and started on the very long and tedious process of rehabilitative therapies. He learned to sit and then to walk. Every day she prepared salmon, his favorite dish, and brought it to him. She would nurture him back. He was struggling to sleep, and then, when given medications to help, he would sleep in the day and struggle to get through his therapies. She began to research natural aides to help with sleep. She brought him tart cherry juice to try to help. She fed him, held him, and talked to him. He would stare blankly, but she told herself, "He is in there, he will be back."

The first crack in her protective shield of denial occurred one day during his speech therapy. As Sissy sat in the session, Roger began to speak, but the words made no sense. He was suffering from visual agnosia, which is the inability to recognize common objects and understand the meaning, name, or use of these objects, and it had been caused by damage to the parietal and temporal lobes of his brain. It also became apparent during the sessions that he suffered from aphasia, or the inability to express or understand common language, both verbal and written.

In other words, it was becoming increasingly clear that Roger did not recognize, know, or understand her. He had no comprehension of the concept of a wife.

This was a new pain and fear to face. Sissy longed and prayed for the day when she would hear his voice once again, the day when he would say her name and hold her as he had for so many years. But this did not happen. His words made no sense, and at times they were even hurtful—a stark contrast to the loving, kind, and funny man she knew. Fear and doubt about his return began to seep into her awareness. But the gravity of those thoughts was too heavy to bear. She pushed them from her mind and replaced them with more numbers and statistics about recovery from traumatic brain injury, more musings over which of his favorite foods to bring him, and more prayers.

Suspending the Present to Manage the Pain

Just as Roger's clinical numbers—blood pressure, intracranial pressure—became Sissy's way of existence, so dates and the passage of time fell out of her awareness. When she and I talked together almost three years after the injury, she acknowledged that dates had been lost for her. With tears running down her face, she admitted that she still did not want to catalogue time or events because she was waiting for her husband to get better and share them with her. She added, "I feel like time just stopped for me. I stopped living, and dates and times didn't matter. I would tell myself that I will catch Roger up on everything when he is home. I simply didn't want to experience living, as nothing mattered without him."

They pushed on as a family. Once Roger was more alert, they began to bring in pictures from family vacations and events to try to spark a memory or connection. Sissy pointed out to me the pictures on the wall in the hallway of their house. "We would take each of these pictures down and take them to the hospital; one by one, we would show him. We hoped they would spark a memory, bring a smile of recognition—anything to bring him back." I walked down the hallway and looked at the pictures. There was a large photo of Roger in an inner tube floating on a lazy river, smiling, with his arms stretched out and the kids pushing him. There was a picture of him holding Race when he was a baby. There was a striking photo of a black-tie event, with Sissy in a beautiful black gown and Roger in his tuxedo, snuggled into each other. The wall was covered from floor to ceiling with memories, reminders of their life as a family. Sissy shared stories with me about each of the photos—she laughed and cried as she thought about the memories. As she lowered herself to the floor, she said, "I can't bring myself to take them off the wall." It was clear that at this juncture she was letting go and beginning to grieve, while still fighting the thought that the Roger on the wall was gone. She wasn't ready to quit. In a way, he was still there in the house; I could feel his presence, and I knew they could as well.

The family's visits to see Roger continued, and each time the children would try to connect with him. He looked like Dad. He was familiar to them. Now if they could just find a way to make themselves familiar to him. Race would talk about basketball—a topic Dad loved. He would tell his father about his basketball practice, about a shot that he had made during the game. But Rogers's lack of response often led to hurt feelings. Race tried to be funny, to make silly jokes that Dad would get and appreciate. There was no response, but he kept trying. Race admitted that his Mom's words rang in his head: "We can love him back because we are his family." He would swallow hard and keep trying with a new topic or new story.

Throughout the visits, Sissy would snap pictures of the kids standing and sitting near Roger's bed as they tried to communicate with him. She thought that someday, when he was better, she would show him the pictures. She would tell him how they had brought him back from his injury, how they had loved him back to them. But when she shared the pictures with me, what I saw was the fear on Siena's face and the mixture of sadness and anger on Race's. They seemed to know before Sissy that the Dad they had loved was gone and would not be coming back. They had begun their own private and painful journey of grieving. And they feared that maybe they would lose their mother too, as they saw how much she was physically declining and heard her crying each day in the shower. They were helpless to fix the situation.

Sissy and her children lived with chronic anxiety—anticipating the next terrible event. While fear is the body's normal and healthy warning signal for danger, anxiety is the cognitive interpretation of how we see a situation and the assessment of our ability to cope with it. After a traumatic experience, the mind often goes into overdrive and becomes hypervigilant, anticipating the next crisis or trauma. Sissy and her children found themselves in a constant state of being on guard, never letting themselves relax and absorb the present. They were living with the fear of the future, anticipating when the next shoe would drop. It was time to conquer the fear by taking control—but in a different way.

CHAPTER 5

Our Destiny Is in Our Control

"In the end, only three things matter: how much you
loved, how gently you lived, and how gracefully you let
go of things not meant for you."

— Buddha

CONTROL IMPLIES MANY things, but it is defined as having power over something. As a psychological concept, it can originate either internally or externally. Individuals who have an external locus or place where their control comes from tend to think that luck or others determine their success or suffering. They are prone to blame others or circumstances, and they often feel powerless. In comparison, those with an internal locus of control believe that they are the source of their own success and have control over their own destinies. They are less likely to be influenced by the opinions of others and often feel more confident when dealing with obstacles.

Individuals with an internal locus of control tend to rely actively on gratitude, according to studies performed by Professor Philip Watkins, from Eastern Washington University. He found that people with an internal source of control acknowledged that others can contribute to their well-being but that, ultimately, they are responsible for how they feel. Actively practicing a life of gratitude increases our joy, life satisfaction, and ability to be resilient and cope.

In an exercise called Gratitude Night, Martin Seligman, a psychology professor at the University of Pennsylvania, asked his class to think about somebody who had made a difference in their lives but whom they had never had a chance to thank. They were instructed to write down how they felt about that person. The person was then invited to join the student in class the next month, without being told why. Standing in front of the class with his or her guest, each student read the testimonial of thanks aloud, and the guest was then presented with the testimonial on a laminated sheet as a gift. The emotion of expressing gratitude and observing others do the same left everyone in the class moved to tears and prompted Seligman to suggest using this gratitude exercise to build authentic happiness.

While this seems like a simple exercise, it is often difficult to push through embarrassment and excuses in order to express gratitude directly. Nevertheless, actively engaging in acts of gratitude builds our strength to battle through pain and tragedy—it is the antidote to suffering. Research has shown that individuals who live intimately with gratitude before trauma strikes are better equipped to cope and thrive after catastrophic events.

Last year, I was invited to give a talk to a group of leaders at an international company on the topic of gratitude and its effect on the financial bottom line. The program addressed how gratitude in the workplace leads to a more engaged and productive workforce. I shared with the group the value of using the gratitude exercise to increase gratitude awareness among the leadership team. Several months after the talk, I received a letter from a woman named Cynthia who had been in the audience. She told me that she had identified her second-grade teacher as somebody who had made a difference in her life and that she had decided to express her gratitude. Cynthia found her former teacher living in an assisted-living senior community, where she met her for lunch. After they had eaten, she read her testimonial letter to her teacher:

When I was a little girl, my mother drank a lot and many times would not wake up early enough to get me to school. My father would fight with her but at the end of first grade I had missed so much school that there was discussion about making me repeat the grade. I don't know if you knew all of that. I know you realized that I was not able to read as well as my classmates and math was very difficult for me.

I always felt nervous and embarrassed in school until I met you. I remember my first day of second grade, walking in your room. You smiled at me and told me you liked my dress. Isn't it funny how I remember that compliment this many years later? But you were so kind to me and when I didn't know an answer you never made me feel stupid. Instead you would work with me privately and always whispered that you thought I was smart. Nobody had ever said that to me. I couldn't wait to get to school each day. I remember praying at night that my mom would wake up on time so I wouldn't miss school and seeing you.

I recently attended a seminar where I was asked to think about somebody who made a difference in my life and I thought about you. I know I was too young then to understand the impact that you had on my life and certainly too young to thank you. But now I want you to know that I have a Master's degree in business and I am a VP of a bank. I hope that makes you proud.

When I struggled in college with classes or felt inadequate in jobs, I thought about you. I remembered you saying that I was smart. You believed in me and made me believe in myself. I am so grateful that you were my teacher. Thank you.

Cynthia's former teacher cried as she listened to these words and said that she had no idea that she had had such an influence on Cynthia. The experience was emotional and transformative for Cynthia. She told me that the experience forced her to focus more on her thoughts—the ones she says to herself and to others. The power of simply saying thank you or acknowledging somebody's contribution has led to improvements in her work and family life.

During crises or stressful times, relying on gratitude may actually be the lifeline we cling to for survival. It is not about feeling grateful but about actively being grateful—which is a choice we consciously make. Gratitude does not remove the pain or intensity of loss, but it does give us the power to gain control over our thoughts and make strategies for coping with trauma. A grateful perspective allows us to focus on what is in our control, as opposed to the events or circumstances that are out of our control. Gratitude has the power to heal us and wake us from a state of simply existing without truly living.

Stefani Schaefer—Sissy—was about to experience this wake-up call.

Dependence Is Not a Bad Word

For almost a year after Roger's accident, Sissy and the kids went to work and school but then would return to the safety of their home. Evenings would be spent with just the three of them cuddled on the couch watching movies. The days of adventure, travel, and fun seemed to be over. There was no energy left to plan a trip, no interest in smiling and making conversation in social settings, and certainly no desire to enjoy life. They were all so wounded that surviving the days and getting strength from each other was all they could manage. The months continued to come and go as they privately grieved their loss.

One day, as a friend watched Sissy feed their many animals and the kids while simultaneously taking a call from the producer of her show to discuss an upcoming segment, she asked, "Don't you feel burned out?" Sissy vividly remembers that moment in the kitchen. The words hit her hard—not because she hadn't felt burned out and exhausted before that but because she hadn't allowed herself to admit it. When she heard the words spoken out loud, the emotional floodgates opened and she began to sob. Both she and her friend were taken aback by what seemed like an extreme reaction to a simple question. Sissy eased herself to the kitchen floor, and her friend wrapped her arms around her and held her. This was the first time that Sissy acknowledged to herself that she was, in fact, overwhelmed and not capable of managing alone. Admitting it, however, made her feel like a failure. Many of us think that we can do it all, fix it all, manage it all—and when we can't, feelings of inadequacy creep in. We hear the silent message that we so often repeat to ourselves: strong women should be able to do it all, and asking for help is a sign of weakness.

The truth of Sissy's new reality was crushing her. She didn't have a partner to pick up the slack. There was nobody to fix the broken exhaust fan in the kitchen while she made dinner or drive the kids to activities while she cleaned. She felt as if she were on a merry-go-round that wouldn't stop. She needed to keep moving. The truth was she was alone, and that thought left her feeling scared, inadequate, and angry. Angry at herself for not being able to do it all, and angry at Roger. Why hadn't Roger taken precautions? Why had he been careless? Why had he let this happen? Why had he left her alone? The anger finally came rushing out.

Her friend held her and gently suggested that it was time to begin constructing a new life—one without Roger. It was time to live again, no matter how frightening the idea might be. Deep down, Sissy knew she was right, and she committed to taking the first step. But the thought left her emotionally exhausted.

Sissy would not only have to wear big-girl shoes but many different hats. She didn't know how she could provide both the light-hearted comic relief that had been Roger's gift and her own sensible, safety-conscious voice for the family. The answer would come in her willingness to rely on support from others, which ultimately is what makes us all stronger and more resilient—indeed, it sustains us.

While it may seem counterintuitive to what we often hear about self-reliance and independence, the fact is that we are not self-sufficient beings. We exist because others exist—our very survival depends on our connections to each other. But it is particularly difficult for women to ask for and accept support from others. We tend to feel diminished and inadequate when we depend on others. This is where gratitude comes in. It opens the door and gives us permission to see support from others as a gift that we should feel proud of, as we welcome reciprocity. Gratitude is actually a sign of strength and independence.

Robert Emmons in his book *Thanks!* argues that to truly know gratitude we must acknowledge our dependence on others to give us what we cannot give ourselves. Our emotional and physical well-being depends on our ability to see interdependence as a gift that makes us stronger, as opposed to something that diminishes us. The challenge, of course, is to bulldoze over the guilt we feel when we acknowledge our need for help.

The Storm of Guilt

Simply walk into the self-help section of any bookstore or library, and you will find ample books for women: how we can overcome the confidence gap, strategies to lean in and succeed, how to find balance in work and life, techniques to work more efficiently, how to raise strong children. Why do we need so many books filled with great advice? Perhaps because culturally women receive very clear, unspoken messages about what it means to be a woman—and yet our roles in work and life often run counter to those messages.

Be strong and ambitious, and climb the work ladder of success. Nurture your children and never miss an after-school event or dinnertime. Be strong and confident. Don't be bitchy or bossy. Ask for the raise or promotion you deserve. Don't be arrogant. Successful women attend after-work events and network. Absent mothers contribute to poorly adjusted children. It is no wonder that we need books to help us navigate these discrepancies and our guilt over not doing things right. We seek guidance through books, lectures, and stories from other women.

Guilt, defined as a feeling of remorse for some offense, real or imagined, that we have committed, typically comes storming in when we feel that we have not lived up to our own or others' expectations. Our voice of inadequacy pounds away when we fail to keep a clean home, raise great kids, climb to the top of the career ladder, make time to connect with friends, or serve as caregivers for every generation in the family.

Certainly some guilt is necessary, to guide us in our moral decisions, and it is through remorse that we learn to correct and heal wrongs we have committed. But when we disproportionately experience guilt, it interferes with our self-worth and leads to shame.

Not only does guilt come from our assessment of the things we are supposed to do but don't, it also comes from the belief that we are ultimately responsible for the behavior of others. That burden leads to the most toxic build-up of guilt. We believe that if our children misbehave, engage in criminal acts, or struggle with mental health, it is our fault. Society reinforces this belief that we—as the mothers, the women, the care-providers—are to blame. Women in leadership positions who leave early to attend a child's softball game are often held accountable for their supposedly poor work ethic, while at the same time they are blamed for neglecting their family, leading to a lonely spouse and unruly children. A woman can also be blamed for aggressive behavior while what she was wearing and how she was behaving become the focus of why she was raped or abused. Blame. Blame. Blame. Guilt. Guilt. Guilt.

The best strategy for coping with life, particularly in the face of trauma and crises, is to accept what is ours and to step out of what does not belong to us. The truth is that we will never achieve balance or perfection, despite our best efforts. Balance is a transient and ever-changing state, which exists only fleetingly. Choosing what we will and will not expend our thoughts on is how we differentiate between healthy and unhealthy guilt. When guilt guides us to be more compassionate and forgiving, we win. When guilt stems from voices telling us what others want, expect, and need from us, it should be replaced with defiance.

Sissy's guilt was coming at her from many directions. She felt guilty for not being able to bring Roger back, for the level of despair her children were living with, for not cooking nutritious meals, for disappointing viewers who continued to pray for Roger, and for her own thoughts as she considered a life without Roger. What would the community think of her? What did she think of herself for letting go of him? The challenge was to face her guilt by correcting and disputing her negative and self-deprecating thoughts, while holding tight to her optimism—the seed for resilient coping.

Grieving without Saying Goodbye

Grieving the death of a loved one is a physical, emotional, and social process. Each of the world's cultures follows rituals for honoring a life and saying good-bye to a person who has passed away. They may involve dressing and viewing the body, burial procedures, and inviting friends and family to celebrate and reminisce about the person's life. In most cultures, food is brought to the family to offer comfort and support. By contrast, however, when somebody is gone but still alive, the grieving process is private, with no true end or plan for how to "move on" in life.

Roger had sustained a traumatic brain injury that left him with no memory of his family, limited functional abilities, and changes in his mood and personality due to the area of the brain that was damaged. The Roger that his family had known and loved was gone; only his body remained. In the weeks after the accident, friends, neighbors, and fans all provided support for Sissy and her family. Many brought in meals, car-pooled the children, and offered personal emotional support to Sissy. Her fans and viewers offered prayers and support. But day-to-day life for Sissy and her children was a never-ending grieving process with no resolution. There was no funeral service to demarcate the final farewell. Instead, Sissy and her children were living a trapped life of painful solitude. Life was moving on despite their desire to turn back time. Guilt, remorse, and sadness filled them whenever they thought about the prospect of continuing without Roger. Sissy later told me, "I knew we could not sustain the kind of life we were living, but I was so afraid of letting go of hope—of him. I prayed for guidance. This aspect of my personal life was now very public, with many kind people praying and supporting me. What would they think? But when I looked into the faces of my children, I knew we had no choice."

Wayne Dawson, Sissy's co-anchor and dear friend, thinks a lot about the strength it takes every day for his friend to keep living her life—raising her children and battling with impossible life choices. As a public figure, Sissy continues to receive emails, letters, and messages from people offering advice, support, criticism, and opinions. However, Wayne is quick to point out that unless people have walked in her shoes, they can't possibly know her pain and therefore should not sit in judgment on her choices. When I spoke with him about the situation, he said, "I was there, and I saw her raw pain—I knew her life would never be the same."

It is still hard for Wayne to think about that day—that moment. During our conversation, he choked up as he remembered guiding Sissy back to see Roger for the first time at the hospital. Looking up at the ceiling, he told me, "It was like nothing I had ever seen before—Roger on that gurney and the look on Sissy's face when she first saw him. I knew, in that moment, that this was out of our hands, and I started to pray silently as I physically held Sissy up." The images still flash through his mind. "I pray for her and the children every day that they will find the strength and courage to make the hard choices and live life," he said.

Sissy knew hard choices had to be made, but any thought of letting go unleashed intolerable pain. What she didn't fully realize was that simply existing was creating its own unbearable sorrow for her family. She was about to witness it.

About a year after Roger's catastrophic fall, Sissy and the kids were riding home from Race's basketball game. The sun was shining, and there wasn't a cloud in the sky. It was quiet in the car—their new normal. Suddenly the silence was broken by screaming and crying coming from the back seat. Race, now a middle-schooler, was yelling: "I hate my life! I want to die. Dear God, why don't you just kill me!" He sobbed and wailed, making loud gasping sounds.

Siena unbuckled her seatbelt and slid over to her brother's side of the car. She grabbed him and started to cry too. "Don't say that—please—please!" she yelled. Sissy recalled feeling as if she had been punched in the stomach—she could hardly catch her breath. "My God, where is this coming from?" she wondered. "Why is he saying this?" She began to panic as she found a side street and pulled the car over.

It was at that moment that Sissy woke up from her terrible nightmare. She was fully aware of herself and her kids for the first time since the call had come about Roger's accident. She took a deep breath, dried her tears, and felt a new sensation wash over her: she felt calm and in control. This took her by surprise. With the car safely parked, she jumped out of the driver's seat, opened the door to the backseat, and slid in next to Race. She took a long look at her kids—really looked at them. They appeared exhausted, lost, and incredibly sad. Of course she knew how hard it had been on them, but only in that moment did she actually feel the depth of their fear and despair. They had lost the father they loved, the man who had made them feel loved and safe, who had made them laugh. And now they feared that they were losing their mother too. Although she was physically present for them, she had known that she was only capable of half-listening to them, as her mind continued to focus on micro-managing Roger's care. She had known that she wasn't taking care of herself and that her physical and emotional decline was evident. However, until that moment she hadn't realized the raw fear that her appearance and their daily life was creating in her children.

Sissy stepped into that moment and took control. She knew she could not change their past or even control what was in their future, but she could control how they managed in the present. She pulled her children into her arms, and they all cried—deep, hard sobs. Then she moved them gently back from her and looked each of them in the eye. She said, "I am sorry. We are our family now. I realize now what maybe both of you already know. We can't make Dad better. What happens to Dad now is out of our hands and in God's hands." They held each other, and Sissy prayed out loud, "God, please wrap your arms around Roger and let him feel that we are loving him." Through his tears, Race looked up at her and smiled. It was a turning point for all three of them.

That day, in the backseat of the car, the family began to say their good-byes to the husband and father they had known. They let go of the need for control that they had been holding onto for so many months, and by doing so they actually felt more in control. The increased immediacy in her thoughts, emotions, and decisions gave Sissy a new feeling of hope. It was not the hope that she had been holding onto before—that Roger would one day recognize them, that he would return home, and that they would be a family again. Instead, in that moment, she consciously and deliberately created a new hope—hope in their survival.

Hope is not an emotion that we experience, and we are not born with it. We create hope through our thoughts and actions. It is a learned strategy for tolerating our disappointments and pain and for coaching ourselves through them. Hope rises from our ability to tap into our inner source of control. The belief that we ultimately control our destiny is how we deal with situations that are out of our control.

As Sissy got back behind the wheel of the car and drove home, she felt peace—a peace she had not felt since that morning when she stood in her gold-heeled, leopard-print, sling-back pumps, kissing Roger good-bye as he left for work. As she glanced in the rearview mirror, she saw relief on the faces of her children. The guilt, anger, fear, and responsibility that they had been bearing had all lifted. They were finally free to begin the grieving process.

Starting a New Life

The first opportunity for the family to leave the safe haven of their home and step out into the social world without Roger was just around the corner. The Fourth of July was approaching, and Sissy knew that their neighbors would be hosting their traditional annual party. Every previous year, Roger, Sissy, and the kids had attended. She knew the routine. Everyone would bring something to share; there would be games, lots of laughter, and fireworks. It was an all-day event that the family looked forward to every year.

Sissy and the children had turned down many social invitations since the accident—it had felt emotionally safer to remain at home with each other and their memories. But Sissy knew that they could not sustain that existence. They would need to face a life with activities and events without Roger. She knew it was the right thing for the kids, though her soul was not ready. She would have to dig deep to find the energy and will to attend.

She smiled sadly as she told me in our interview that getting ready for the party had been exhausting. "I put on an outfit and then would change. I had such a knot in my stomach that made it so hard to breath. It seems like such a simple thing, to go to a party with friends that I know and love. But deep down I knew it was the beginning of my new life without him. It was as if, going to that party, I was admitting to myself that he wasn't coming back. I so didn't want to face that reality." As she spoke a tear dripped down her cheek.

When she had finally finished getting dressed, she went downstairs and tried to be cheerful with the children as they packed up the food they were bringing. The kids smiled back but seemed nervous as well. They all realized that it would be their first time participating in a family tradition without being a complete family. Their longing for Roger was intense as they climbed into the car. When Sissy pulled into their friends' driveway, the knot in her stomach tightened. She tried to fight the tears that were forming. She needed to be strong for the kids, she kept reminding herself. The car was quiet as she put it into park, and then came the muted sounds of Siena crying. Nobody said a word. They simply held hands and sat for five, ten, fifteen minutes. After twenty minutes they finally exited the car. Still holding hands, they began to walk up the driveway.

"The driveway seemed so long as I forced a smile on my face to greet our host," Sissy told me. The children separated from her and joined the other kids, who were laughing and dancing to music. Sissy began to make her way through the crowd, hugging and kissing her friends while making smalltalk. Her heart felt heavy, and her parallel thoughts were running again: Roger would really like the pasta salad, Roger would laugh at the way the kids were dancing, Roger...

As she found a spot in the grass and laid her blanket down, Sissy could hear the boom of the fireworks starting. She looked up into the sky at the burst of colors, and a deep loneliness settled over her. She remembered how it had felt when Roger was sitting next to her. How it had felt when he told her how pretty she looked, or that he liked her outfit. How it had felt when he put his hand on the small of her back and guided her into a room, or put his arm around her shoulder and gently pulled her to him. She longed for those familiar feelings. She wondered how many times she had taken them for granted. Then she started to cry: she realized that she was no longer reminding herself to remember the details of the day so that she could someday share with him all that he had missed. The hope of him ever returning to her was gone, and its departure created an intense pain that vibrated through every part of her body.

As her friends approached, she wiped her tears away and shifted these thoughts to the back of her mind. Then, moving into autopilot, she smiled, chatted, and laughed, while the empty feeling inside her settled into that hidden, private place. As the final round of fireworks was released, she and the children waved, smiled, and said their good-byes. They returned home feeling worn out. After the children fell asleep, Sissy climbed into her bed—their bed. She felt exhausted, as if every ounce of strength had been pulled from her. After a moment she rolled over onto Roger's pillow, buried her face, and sobbed. She could no longer smell him on the pillow or feel him in the room. Roger was gone and would not be coming back to their home, to their life, to her. The task was complete—they were now a family of three.

Resilience: The Power to Transform

The emotional resilience to cope and thrive after trauma does not mean that the wound or pain is not present. It does not mean that people "move on" and gain "closure," as if the trauma has been tucked away in some closet. Trauma, pain, and loss permanently change how we think, feel, and react in our lives. But resilience gives us the power to transform our lives as we move through the trauma.

Practicing strategies to learn and sustain resilience begins with a full awareness of how we feel. While it is certainly easier to numb and ignore our feelings in the moment, the reality is that they won't go away. Awareness and acknowledgment of our emotions provide the fuel for action—actively seeking support, reorganizing our thought patterns to facilitate optimism, grabbing control over the things we can influence, and using humor to maintain perspective. Finally, the deepest foundation for resilience is gratitude. The active, conscious choice to live with gratitude gives us the power to integrate pain and joy.

CHAPTER 6

———— ✂ ————

Healing: The Integration of Sadness and Joy

"The two most important days in your life are the day
you were born and the day you figure out why."

— MARK TWAIN

SANDY WAS A petite, fifty-six-year-old woman with short blonde hair and
dark brown eyes that shone even with a weak smile. She was a patient on
the cardiac floor of the hospital where I was working, and she had been
there approximately two months, waiting for her heart-transplant surgery.
Despite a very real threat of death and visible signs that she was losing
her strength each day, she clung to hope. From the start, Sandy would
greet me with a warm smile and a cheerful demeanor. She was more
than willing to talk to me, readily accepting the fact that patients in that
wing were expected to be assessed and followed by a psychologist. She
used our time together to talk about her fear of death and to express her
sadness at the thought of leaving her family. Her loving family was ever-
present in that hospital room; their photos hung on the walls and sat in
frames on the nightstand. They slept in her room at night and kept vigils
in the chairs during the day. She drew strength from them. Outwardly she
remained optimistic and hopeful for their sake.

But during our private time together, Sandy was beginning to let go
of her hope for survival. She was working on her courage so that she
could share her fears and prepare her family for her death, particularly her

twenty-five-year-old daughter, Anne. As Anne was an only child, Sandy wanted to leave her with the pearls of wisdom and guidance that a mother typically shares with her daughter as she prepares to marry. Plans were being made for Anne's wedding, which was only months away. Sandy's dilemma was how to say good-bye and still leave room for the happiness that surrounds getting married and starting a new life. She cried when she talked about this to me. She was clearly beginning to let go of her family and her life.

The only solace for Sandy was her confidence in her daughter's emotional strength and faith. This, coupled with the knowledge that Anne was surrounded by loving friends and family, gave her comfort and the hope that her daughter would be all right after she was gone. Each day, Sandy grew weaker and the family grew more desperate. The end was imminent.

The following Thursday, at about 2:30 am, my pager went off with the message that Sandy was being rushed into surgery—a heart had just arrived.

The cardiac transplant surgery was successful, and Sandy quickly started to regain her strength. The staff called it a miracle. Her family saw her making remarkable progress in her physical recovery, but they also saw that she was emotionally paralyzed. She was not the same person. Their conversations were superficial, and her warm, easy smile was now replaced by a plastic imitation. Intellectually they understood—but they desperately wanted Sandy back. After all, their prayers had been answered. She was alive.

As the months passed, Sandy learned how to smile at happy moments, but in reality she hadn't felt real joy since she had learned the truth about the organ transplanted into her chest. She had convinced herself that feeling happy or joyful would be disrespectful to the heart's previous owner. Nevertheless, on the special day of her daughter's wedding, she found herself caught up in the moment, laughing and smiling. From across the room, her husband saw her joy and choked back a tear: there was the Sandy he loved. He watched her open her mouth wide, letting out a hearty laugh as she watched a little boy dance and spin himself upside down on the dance floor. This little ring-bearer, Jake, was only three years old, but he could certainly cut some moves in his tiny tuxedo. The more she laughed, the more Jake performed. Sandy was painfully aware that this was the first time she had laughed or even allowed herself to smile genuinely since—that day. The day that seemed so long ago, when she had read the headline in the local newspaper and learned the truth about her heart. It was the day when she became somebody else, or when somebody else became her.

Pulling herself from her thoughts, Sandy glanced around the beautiful reception hall and caught a glimpse of the stunning bride, who was smiling back at her. Her daughter was indeed a breathtaking young woman. From across the room, Sandy watched Anne greeting her guests and kissing her new husband as their glasses clinked. She knew how blessed she was to be alive and to be standing there, witnessing the moment, but her mind flashed back again to the words on the front page of the newspaper.

It read, "High School Athlete's Death Gives Life." The car accident had left Tina brain-dead, and her organs were donated and sent to different hospitals across the country, with the exception of her heart, which was sent to the local hospital—the one where Sandy had been waiting for a replacement heart. The news spread that the local high-school's softball coach, who had been on the transplant list for months, received a heart that evening. Although the hospital would not share the clinical information, it did not take long for the logical conclusion to be drawn: Tina's heart had been given to Sandy, her own softball coach.

Tina had been an average athlete—not the strongest or fastest—but she hadn't seemed to mind. She loved playing the game. She could usually be found in the dugout, dumping water on somebody or making jokes to lighten the mood. As the coach for the team, Sandy often thought that with more practice and a better work ethic, Tina could become a better player. But Tina only wanted to have fun and had no desire or talent to play beyond high school.

The article haunted Sandy. Although many people tried to explain it away as a possible coincidence, deep down she knew the truth. She felt it. Now, at the wedding, Anne and her mother shared a knowing look from across the room. Sadness sat quietly behind their smiles. Sandy instinctively turned away, and with a gentle movement placed her hand on her chest—a motion that was now almost as reflexive as a sneeze. Her shimmering silk gown covered her chest from view, but she could still feel the scar. In a light, stroking motion, her hands moved across the long, raised bump in the center of her chest. Then, still following her new routine, she held her hand still and felt the rhythmic beat of the heart. She felt Her. She was beating, rhythmic and steady. Her heart was alive. The young high-school girl who had lived in their town, who had played center field for the high-school softball team, was with them. Tina's heart was beating in Sandy's chest. The tears fell, and guilt returned.

While there are many emotional issues to resolve surrounding the science of organ transplantation, survivor's guilt seems to be the heaviest. Praying for a heart often becomes a troubling burden—patients often express guilt for "praying that somebody would die so I could live." This struggle was certainly present in Sandy's case. Often she asked herself, "Why am I still here when somebody so young is gone? How can I laugh when she cannot? How can I express happiness and be so selfish and disrespectful to her family?" These are the conflicting voices that float in the heads of many survivors, who have benefited from those who are gone, either in body or spirit.

Fighting the Laughter

On January 17th, 2007, in Baghdad, Iraq, a grenade was thrown under the car of a young American woman—a civilian on a peace-keeping mission—and killed her. Far away, in Perry, Ohio, a fourth-grade gym teacher, fifty-seven-year-old Andre Parhamovich, was teaching his class. He laughed hard as he watched one of his young students, the comedian of the class, complete a silly dance move. It was the last time he would laugh without guilt.

Before the class ended, Coach Parhamovich was called to the office to take a phone call. This was an unusual occurrence, and it made him tense up as he walked down the hall toward the reception area, his mind beginning to spin. Was his wife all right? The grandkids? Had his teenage twin boys gotten to school on time?

When we spoke together, much later, Andre looked at me as these memories returned, then dropped his eyes and closed them. Making eye-contact had been difficult for Andre from the first day that he entered my counseling office. It was as if averting his eyes from his surroundings, from others, from life would help him stay numb and disconnected from his pain.

With heavy sobs, he stepped back into the moment and said, "I knew something terrible had happened when I walked into the office and picked up the phone. I remember feeling light-headed—a deep feeling of dread stirred." The voice on the other end of the line confirmed the panic rising inside of him. It was the voice of his daughter Marci, but the connection was poor and his hearing aid was buzzing. He could tell Marci was crying. "I thought I heard her say 'dead,' but the words were hard to hear, or maybe hard to absorb," he said.

Andre quickly handed the phone to the secretary and asked her to take the message. "I can still see the look on her face—pale and staring— as she slowly sat down in her chair and the principal moved closer to her," he told me.

"Is my wife okay? Is Vicky dead?" he yelled at them. The room fell silent, and in that moment he realized. "I don't remember if they said it or if I said it, but the words 'Andi is dead' were echoing in the room," he told me.

His beautiful daughter Andi had been killed in Iraq. The moments that followed were fuzzy, and time moved slowly as he walked down the school hallway to his car. He remembers passing Mrs. Barth, who had been Andi's favorite teacher. She smiled at him and asked if he was okay.

Nausea swept over him, and he ran to his car. "Andi is dead. Her convoy was attacked—they killed her," he recalled his other daughter telling him that day. Talking to me, he could still hear the words clearly in his head.

Andrea Parhamovich—Andi, as her friends and family called her—was a determined, funny, confident young woman who wanted to make a difference in the world. After graduating from Marietta College, she moved to Boston, Massachusetts, and started her career in political communication in the Governor's Office. Her career path then took her to New York City, where she worked for Miramax Films and Air America Radio. But her strong desire to promote democracy led her to join the National Democratic Institute, and she took part in a trip to Iraq to assist with training sessions on strategies to advance democracy.

Her father laid his head back on his chair in my office and continued to sob as his thoughts moved in all directions. He looked at me and said, "I blame myself. I was her father. I was supposed to protect her—to demand that she not go. I don't even remember if I fought with her about going. Did I yell and forbid her? How did she end up there—a place where I couldn't protect her? They targeted her—they wanted to kidnap her. Oh my God, what would they have done to her? Should I be grateful that she was killed instead? She burned to death—oh my God, they burned her! Did she feel it? I pray it was over quickly for her—I dream about it. Her beautiful smile, her laugh and sense of humor—up in flames." His sobbing was harder now, and, with his eyes closed, he did not seem to be aware of anything in the present. I sat still with him.

For eight years, Andre has continued to battle through guilt, despair, and anger. It is a daily struggle. Some days, when he reminisces about walking his little girl to school or watching her play softball, the pain swallows him. Anger comes rushing in when he thinks about how many questions surrounding her death are still unanswered. Why didn't our government protect her? Why was she allowed to enter such a dangerous area of the city? What does our government have to hide? Despair settles over him as he contemplates the fact that he will never walk her down the aisle, hold her babies, or proudly watch all that she would have accomplished in life.

He finds hope and some solace as he walks near the water and sits on a bench that is inscribed with her name: "Andi Parhamovich: Gave her life to promote peace—Now walks with angels." Andre writes letters to his daughter, composes poems to share in his grief support groups, and speaks to others who have lost children; he finds comfort in these acts. Andre knows that time has forced him to move on in life, but it is not the same life. He consciously works hard to find the courage and strength to get out of bed and live a life that would make Andi proud. He thinks The Andi Foundation would make her smile.

The Foundation was established in her memory to give financial support to young women and thus help them achieve their educational aspirations and make a difference in the world. It offers scholarships, housing, and internship programs to help young women grow in leadership and advocacy. Women from many countries have benefited from The Andi Foundation and have returned to their own countries armed with the knowledge and skills to promote change and fight for human rights.

As for the father who lost his daughter in a brutal attack, Andre struggles daily to give himself permission to laugh or feel joy. "There are wonderful things in my life—people and times that make me happy, but guilt seems to quickly turn those feelings off," he told me. "When I get caught up in a moment and I find myself laughing, I immediately feel guilt. It's like a reflex. How can I laugh or feel happy without Andi? It feels so disrespectful to her."

Andre invited me to join him on a visit to Andi's bench. As we sat there, staring at the water, he said, "It is so hard to believe it has been almost eight years—pushing through the pain. But when I sit here, I feel her. I hear her. No, not actual voices," he chuckled. "I know the best way for me to love and remember her is to allow myself to live—to forgive myself and those responsible for her death and to invite laughter and joy back into my life. The joy and laughter is a watered-down version of what I knew before, but at least it is something. I continue to work on giving myself permission to laugh. Now, when I laugh hard, I imagine Andi laughing with me."

Joy and Sadness

Stefani Schaefer—Sissy—understands the guilt of laughing and living. There didn't seem to be a place for joy or fun in her life without her husband, Roger. But sometimes the human spirit knows best and guides us to the discovery that joy can exist in the face of grief, that perhaps the best way to honor those we love who are gone is to carry our grief with us, as we continue to live fully—living with both our tears and our laughter. This truth came to Sissy one beautiful sunny day, on a short weekend trip to the beach that she took with her children.

Sissy sat in the sand as the kids waded into the ocean. She watched them as they were tossed around by the waves. They needed this trip—a time alone with sunshine and each other. The sun was beating down on Race and Siena, and Sissy smiled to herself and thought how much they were changing—growing up. She took a long look at Race as he stood in the water. He was growing tall and handsome just like his father, with the same mannerisms and sense of humor. Siena, with her silly expressions and spirited personality, was a reflection of the light energy that Roger had created in their home. It made her smile as she thought, "I still have the best of Roger with me and always will."

The kids smiled and waved to her. She called out to them, "Jump the waves!" Race and Siena held hands and began to jump and smile. They jumped, fell, laughed, and jumped again. The sun was glistening on their wet bodies, and Sissy felt joy. She yelled to them, "Jump higher," as she pulled her phone out and started snapping pictures. The waves crashed and pulled them as they continued to laugh—really laugh. It was a sound she had not heard for a very long time. Her mind traveled back to the last time she had seen the kids this happy or felt it herself.

Images rose in her mind of crystal-clear, turquoise water splashing on their feet as they jumped waves and posed for pictures on the beach in

Kauai, Hawaii. The whole family wore white pants and tops with matching, black-beaded necklaces. They were celebrating Sissy and Roger's wedding anniversary by returning to the spot where they had exchanged vows fourteen years earlier. As she thought about the trip, she recalled how Roger had planned many fun-filled adventures for them. It was a trip filled with laughter and joy, only a few months before the accident. Now a tear slid down her cheek. That had been only a few years ago, but the sadness that they were all carrying made it feel like a lifetime ago.

They had been holding back on feeling true happiness for such a long time. Such emotions felt out of place in light of their loss. Nobody felt like laughing, and when they did they held back to avoid hurting each other. There were times when Sissy would catch herself laughing and then immediately be struck with guilt and shame. How could she laugh or feel happy ever again when Roger wasn't with them? When she experienced moments of happiness, it felt like a betrayal of him. Most of the time she wasn't even aware that she wasn't allowing herself to smile genuinely or to feel happy.

But she knew that when she let go and truly felt happy, the children would follow. They were watching her and following her lead on how to cry, laugh, and live. For a long time Sissy had understood intellectually that holding back from fully living would not change her circumstances; it would not bring Roger back; all it would do was prevent her and the kids from enjoying their future. They deserved to live fully in the moment—and now she understood this emotionally too.

Sissy turned her attention back to the children jumping in the waves and laughing—laughing hard. Without thinking, she found herself on her feet, running toward the water. This time as she ran her legs felt light. Time moved with her. She felt the moment—the wind in her hair, the sand under her feet, and the warmth of the sun on her face. She ran faster. She handed her phone to a woman sitting nearby and asked if she would take their picture. Running into the water, she took her children's hands and jumped as the next wave came crashing in. They laughed and smiled and for the first time since the accident actually experienced joy.

As they boarded the plane to return home, Sissy felt lighter: not only had her energy changed, but her perspective was different. She had found clarity. She reached across the aisle and grabbed Siena's hand, squeezing it as they both smiled. Their mood remained cheerful during the car-ride home from the airport. The car was filled with laughter, chatter, and smiles—and the smiles were natural and easy, stripped of the weight of guilt that had tied them down for so long. Sissy dropped the kids off at a friend's house for the afternoon and stopped at the drug store to print the pictures of their day at the beach. She was eager to see on paper what she knew she had felt the day before.

As she pulled into her driveway and parked the car in the garage, she sat for a moment. Her stillness made a stark contrast to the routine that she had created for herself—a routine of constant motion to avoid absorbing her new reality. Of course, her schedule was often tight now, as a single mother, but she also knew that staying busy and distracting herself was easier—emotionally safer. Now, things were changing. She sat in her car for a while and then slowly forced her eyes to look out the window at Roger's car, parked next to hers. She had been keeping up the general maintenance on it, wanting it to be in good condition when he returned home and needed to drive it. Maybe, deep down, she had known before that he would not be coming home and would never drive his car again. But it wasn't until this moment that she allowed the thought to become conscious. She took a deep breath and got out of her own car. Then she placed her hand gently on the hood of his car and lowered her head.

Stepping into the house, she put her suitcase down near the stairs. Instead of running up the steps and quickly unpacking, starting a laundry, and sorting the mail, she walked into the living room and forced herself to take in the silence. Only now, several years after that morning when she had laughed with Roger and said good-bye as he walked out the door, could she bring herself to say her final good-bye. She slowed her mind and her body down, sat on a dining-room chair, and took a good look around the room. It was an act that she tended to avoid by keeping herself busy and focused on tasks. The crowded routine of her life had kept her distracted from her pain, her loss, her new reality—but that too was changing.

She looked around the room; Roger's presence could be seen and felt everywhere. There was the wall covered in crucifixes that they had collected on their many trips. Each cross held a memory. She whispered a little prayer and then turned her attention to the fish tank that Roger had skillfully placed inside the wall of the dining room. She remembered the day when he had cut through the tiles in the kitchen to complete the wiring; they had all clapped when the first fish were placed inside the tank. Moving her gaze past the fish tank into the kitchen, she glanced at the hardwood floor and the color swatches that were still leaning against the wall—the project of refinishing the floor had been about to begin before the accident. Roger had wanted the darker color, and Sissy was partial to the lighter shade. The final decision had never been made.

Her eyes moved to the pictures of him on the walls and the end tables. There were photos of him with his arms around her, smiling, holding Siena in the hospital as a newborn baby. Her favorite picture showed him laughing as he danced with her on the beach in Hawaii. "He will always be with us," she thought.

Her gaze moved to a beautiful etched-glass bowl on a table in the corner, now covered in dust. Inside the bowl were countless wine corks, on which she and Roger had written many different things over the years. Some had the dates of special occasions, some reminded her of places they had been, some had a short story about what they were doing, and some had intimate messages for each other. Each one of the corks represented a part of her life with him. Before the accident, Roger had sometimes dumped them out on the floor so that the two of them could read them and laugh, cry, and reminisce about old moments. Sissy reached in and pulled out one of the corks. She smiled as she read the message, and her tears flowed. The handwriting was his, and the memory was theirs. She had a fleeting thought of taking the cork with her the next time she went to see him, but instead she slipped the cork back into the bowl. The

Roger that she now visited would not understand the message or remember the memory—that Roger was gone.

Her relationship with him had ended without her permission, desire, or control. She knew that it was time for her to accept her new reality and say good-bye to Roger. She had been grieving for several years but had never given herself permission to let him go. Slowly she emptied the bowl of corks—the bowl filled with meaningful dates, shared memories, and intimate messages—onto the floor. Then she poured herself a glass of wine, just as they had when they were together. Sitting cross-legged on the floor, she began reading, laughing, reminiscing, and remembering. Hours passed before she realized that it was getting late and that the kids would soon be coming home.

Later, when she was speaking with me, she smiled as she remembered scooping up all the corks and placing them back in the beautiful bowl. "They are my reminders, my memories of my Roger," she told me. She reached in her purse and pulled out the photos of her and her children jumping in the waves. "Look at their faces," she said. "They—no we—were so happy in that moment." She reached into a drawer, pulled out a frame, and placed one of the photos into it. She smiled as she took a black marker and wrote on the bottom of the picture, "The moment it was okay to jump for joy." She hung the picture in their bathroom.

Now they all smile when they look at this picture. Roger would love it too, for the very essence of him was about living—really living. He was a free spirit who would be proud that his family has found a way to jump and embrace the joy of life again.

The Chinese character for "crisis" is a combination of two words that loosely translate into "danger" and "opportunity." Now, I know that those who have suffered tremendous sorrows would be hard-pressed to swallow the notion that something positive—an opportunity—could arise from their pain. And many would argue they wouldn't welcome it in any case. To say that things happen for a reason and that good comes from trauma would be grossly unfair and disrespectful to those who have lived through pain and loss. Instead it seems reasonable to say that trauma changes us—and in our battle to survive the pain, we need to reach out beyond ourselves for opportunities to convert our pain into help for others.

In the face of unthinkable tragedy and loss, and with the support of her family, friends, community, and faith, Sissy discovered the gift of absorbing the moments of life. Although she has always been known as a positive and compassionate person, she admits that her biggest surprise since the tragedy has been the joy and serenity that she now feels at a deep level. Bravely, she now steps into each moment to confront the joy with the pain. It is the hidden gift.

PART III

Empathy:
The Courage to Walk in
the Shoes of Another

CHAPTER 7

Survival: #76244

SHE ANSWERED THE phone on the third ring. The tone of her voice was soft and low, with a rhythmic cadence to her words that was almost hypnotic. As I held the phone close to my ear, I could feel my heart-rate slow and the volume of my voice lower to mirror hers. I felt relaxed in a strange way. She agreed to an interview and graciously invited me to her home in Florida for a conversation.

During the plane-ride, I closed my eyes and tried to imagine an interview with one of the few remaining Holocaust survivors from Schindler's list. Rena Ferber Finder had agreed to share her story with me. In the weeks prior, I had read and watched numerous videos about the Holocaust. With shame and embarrassment, I had discovered that despite my combined twenty-one years of formal education, this was the first time that I was really learning much about that time in our history. Of course, like most of us, I knew the facts and had seen the horrible images, but I had never really been challenged to think morally or ethically about the real issues that were present then and now. It was Margot Stern Strom, the founder of Facing History and Ourselves, who suggested that if I really wanted to understand and talk about empathy in a meaningful way, a conversation with Rena would be enlightening.

A Holocaust survivor was not on my radar when I set out to interview and talk to women about success. But throughout this journey, I have been learning to reconstruct my thoughts about what success means, apart from achievements, fame, and awards. I have heard and pondered the stories of women who, through their perseverance and courage, have breathed new life for me into words like "grace," "gratitude," and "the power of empathy."

These are not just words for Rena. As a survivor of the Holocaust, she needed to cling with all her strength to these concepts for her survival. Simple acts of compassion and empathy—those she experienced and those she imagined—are why she is alive today.

The Brain Is Wired for Empathy

The human brain has 100 billion neurons or nerve cells, and each neuron can connect or communicate with 10,000 other neurons, yielding an astonishing minimum of 100 trillion synaptic connections or pathways for communication. We actually have the power to create connective pathways through repetition—in essence, we can create our own brain. And empathy is one of the pathways that we can strengthen or diminish through our actions.

It turns out that our brains are actually wired to be empathic. We are neurologically equipped with the ability to feel what others feel, to see what they see, and to view the world through their experiences. This is accomplished through something called "mirror neurons," which give us the ability to step into another person's shoes. It is an involuntary process that allows us to know what another person is feeling and feel it ourselves. We can experience shame, disgust, fear, and compassion by simply watching the experiences of another. It is why we cry when we read the story of somebody in distress and why, when we watch a movie with bugs crawling around, we feel them on our skin. The neural networks of the brain recreate the feelings in us as observers. We become empathic.

Empathy requires imagination and a willingness to enter the emotional state of another. But this process takes courage and attention, for it is hard to un-hear, un-see, and un-know what is now in your awareness. It is easier to block out the suffering and need in others from the beginning. Turning away later is harder—though, sadly, not impossible. Our cognitive brain does have the ability to override this exquisitely intuitive system by using distractions and providing intellectual justifications for choosing to ignore others.

Research clearly demonstrates that when we are distracted by daily tasks, such as reading emails, scanning our phones, replaying an argument with a partner, or simply running through a to-do list, we become less aware of others. We short-circuit the neuronal connections, step out of the awareness of our immediate surroundings, and thus weaken the connections. In other words, our powers of empathy are subject to a "use it or lose it" phenomenon. If empathic neuronal connections sit dormant, they can be lost, and we then become numb to others and ourselves. We risk losing our empathy and thus setting in motion a cascading effect of self-destruction and isolation. Empathy is best strengthened through neurologically experiencing the stories of others. It is nurtured by living with gratitude and courageously stepping into knowing things that we may not want to know—particularly about ourselves. Empathy provides the mirror by which we can honestly and accurately see ourselves.

During my flight to Florida, I was keenly aware of the apprehension I was feeling at the thought of meeting Rena and hearing her story. I knew it would take compassion and courage to step into her world. Fears about the unknowns of that world and about my own possible reactions were rising within me as I pulled into her driveway in Delray Beach.

Rena greeted me at the door with a smile and a warm hug. She stood just a little over five feet tall, with sandy-colored hair that in the sunlight showed strawberry tones. Her brilliantly colored shirt was a mosaic of different shades of sea glass—teals, vibrant blues, and warm streaks of black that brightened her complexion. Although her smile was kind, I could see that, behind her wire-rimmed glasses, her gray eyes held a film of sadness.

She welcomed me into her home and suggested that we "get to know each other before we begin the interview." She guided me into her kitchen, where she was preparing our lunch. The kitchen was cheery, with bright colors and natural light streaming in through the many windows.

At the age of eighty-six, Rena moved slowly and deliberately. With gentle care she washed the grapes and prepared the sandwiches.

An hour passed as we sat at the small kitchen table, sharing lunch and stories about our families. Rena talked about her husband, Mark Finder, also a Holocaust survivor, who had passed away just the previous year. She admitted that there had been a "quiet connection" between them because of their shared experiences—but, she quickly added, they never spoke of them. "It was too painful and frightening to open up the raw wounds with each other," she explained. Her voice trailed off as she recalled her husband's final days. "Before he took his last breath, he told me that his father was coming to get him in a car. His father would save him… He saw his father coming. He seemed at peace, and that gave me peace." She added, "It is what most of us turn to when we are afraid, you know, a deep expectation and hope that our parents will protect us—save us." Her eyes lowered, and she looked hard at her plate; a memory was clearly stirring. She pushed it away and suggested that we move into the living room.

The walls of the living room were covered in family photos that revealed four generations: their three children, six grandchildren, and two great-grandchildren. Rena took one picture off the wall and gently stroked it. The picture showed a smiling woman holding her children. "This is my daughter," she whispered. "I lost her to cancer several years ago. Some losses you never get over." She replaced the photo on the wall and then smiled and pointed to a photo of herself with Academy-Award-winning filmmaker Steven Spielberg. The photo had been taken at the United Nations, where they had both spoken at the International Day of Commemoration in Memory of the Victims of the Holocaust. Spielberg directed the movie "Schindler's List," a story of the genocide of Jews in World War II and the efforts of Oskar Schindler, a war profiteer who saved over a thousand Jews from the gas chamber. Rena has developed a deep friendship with Mr. Spielberg. "He is a brave and kind man to have told the story through his incredible movie. It opened people's eyes to what actually happened," she said.

As I set up the camera and positioned the chairs for our interview, there was a perceptible shift in the atmosphere of the room. It was as if we had entered a sacred place, in which casual conversation was no longer appropriate or welcome. I took my seat across from her, reached over, and turned on the camera and microphone. I was aware of the anxiety that was settling over me in the quiet room. I felt as if I were entering a dark cave, and I became more and more certain that I was ill-prepared for what I might witness. But Rena didn't seem to notice my hands shaking or my shifting in the chair. She seemed to be no longer in the bright, safe room at all but rather back in a place of darkness. She sat very still, her eyes seemingly focused on her hands, though clearly her vision was of another scene. The room grew heavy with a thick silence as she took a noticeable deep breath and began to share her story.

I was transported. I didn't simply step into her shoes intellectually, understanding her experience on a rational level. Instead, I found myself standing next to her in the concentration camp, filled with fear and horror. I too had left the safety of her living room. Through my many years as a psychologist, I have known the power of empathy—the ability to feel what another is feeling—but I have never been so swept into another life as I was in that moment. The power of her story—a little girl losing her innocence, her hope, her faith, her very identity—can be truly shared only in Rena's own words.

Did God See #76244?

"It was May. The sky was so blue, and the sun was shining. It was such a welcome change from the cold that we had been enduring. We stood there on the upper plank several hours, waiting for our usual roll. The roll-call process was often a painful and difficult experience to endure—standing in brutal temperatures for hours, with fear making the body so tense. But today the warmth of the sun and clear sky made it more bearable. As I glanced to my right at the view, it still seemed not real to me. There we were—thousands and thousands of us, standing in single lines, waiting to be counted. Counted because we were now simply a number. I was #76244.

"My private thoughts were interrupted by an unusual sound of music. Was I hearing things? Had my sanity finally been lost? The sound grew louder. It was a lullaby. At first played in Polish and then English, and it was coming from the loudspeaker. The song was so out of place given the surroundings. The volume grew louder and louder, and I began to feel an unexplained nausea flood over me. Something was not right. The music felt eerie and so misplaced. I felt my body tense and my heart begin to pound.

"The music continued to play as a voice began to shout over the music. 'We are taking the children to a special school,' the voice said. And the music continued to play as the cries from mothers could be heard—first crying, then hysterical screaming that echoed through the hills. And the lullaby continued to play. The commanding voice shouted again that if anybody moved, the children would be shot. The air was still as nobody moved. The lullaby played on, but louder. The line of ten thousand people was still as if frozen in time. From the place we stood, we could clearly see a new line forming below in the valley. It was a line of guards, marching while holding the hands of little children and carrying babies in their arms.

"The lullaby played. The faces of the children could be seen from where I stood—many were smiling and laughing at the opportunity to be outside in the sunshine. They had been held inside for so long that the fresh air was clearly being enjoyed. They looked happy as the sun was shining on them. They had been told they were going on a picnic, and many were skipping along at the idea. They were happy and excited. The sun beaming down and the blue sky with white clouds were so welcoming. I stood silent and still as I watched the long line of more than three hundred children and babies being carried away by the soldiers. The lullaby continued to ring through the hills as the last of the line disappeared from view.

"There would be no picnic, no special school. The children were being taken to the death camp to be burned. As I stood there with the sun shining down on my face, watching the happy, innocent faces of those children, I remember thinking that the heavens would open up and take them. That the blue sky above me would open and the children would be saved and protected. It did not happen. The sky never opened. The air was heavy, and the lullaby played.

"In that moment, I lost my faith. I didn't believe there was God. I had been taught that there was God. We had prayed as a family to God—but that was before. That was when it was easy to believe there was God. But now, everything was different. We were alone. There was no God with us. We were alone and invisible. Nobody saw us even when they looked at us. Cruelty, constant fear, torture, and impending death were mine to bear alone in the concentration camp— #76244 would stand alone.

"But there was a time when I was a person—just a happy, innocent little girl."

Learning Compassion and Hope

Krakow, in Poland, is a beautiful city with cobblestone streets and architecturally grand buildings lining the Vistula River. Nestled in a valley at the foot of the Carpathian Mountains, the landscape is spectacular. Rena lived next to the ancient castle and across the street from the river. Her community was filled with culture, art, and academics. It was in this town that she was born, on February 24th, 1929, to Moses and Rozia Ferber. Although she was an only child, she never felt lonely. She was surrounded by grandparents, cousins, and other relatives in her beautiful town.

The gifts of self-worth and confidence were given to Rena by her maternal grandmother. "I loved my grandmother. She was the person who nurtured, cuddled, and made me feel special," Rena said. Her grandparents lived right behind their home, and from Rena's balcony in the kitchen she could see right into their kitchen. "I would go out on the balcony and call for my grandmother—sometimes just to come and play with me, but most often I needed her to come to help me with my multiplication table." Rena recalled that her mother was not as patient with her lessons because Rena had many other chores to attend to after school. But her grandmother was always gentle and kind with her. "I see her like it is today, standing on her balcony, smiling and waving to me."

Most days, after school, her grandmother would come over to Rena's house, take her into the bathroom, and close the door. She would take a seat on the toilet as Rena positioned herself on the edge of the tub. Rena's math lesson would then begin. Her grandmother was patient and kind throughout the lesson—smiling, nodding, encouraging Rena when she struggled. "She would tell me I was smart as she stroked my long braided hair. It was our special time," Rena told me with a smile. Her grandmother taught Rena not only math but the power of self-worth and compassion—gifts that would give Rena the strength to stand up for herself and others in the years that followed.

Rozia, Rena's mother, was a hardworking, strong, cheerful, and resourceful woman who taught Rena to sew, cook, and be kind to others. "My mother was a very smart woman who never complained," Rena said. She possessed a vigilant competence and kept the household and their daily lives in order with her practical and well-structured routines. In the end, these skills proved to be survival skills that helped to save her and Rena.

Rena flashed me a sad smile. "Even as the guards were forcing us to leave our home, my mother was instructing me to scrub the floor and tidy up the apartment. I remember, back then, thinking how odd the request was." Now, when Rena remembers the armed guards outside their door, their bags being packed, and her on her knees scrubbing the floor, she thinks that perhaps it was her mother's way of trying to keep normality, routine, and hope alive. She remembers her mother saying, "We want the place to be ready for us when we return." But after years of deep reflection, Rena has come to believe that her mother was simply trying to distract her daughter from seeing the fear in her own eyes. Rena's mother was strong, and from that day forward she was always on her guard, avoiding her emotions and focusing on her one goal—to protect Rena.

Still, it was Rena's father who ultimately kept her sane during her time in hell, by teaching her about hope. Rena described her father as a loving man with a strong faith. When she talked about him to me, she smiled with a deep, warm glow. "He believed in the good of people," she said, then quietly added, "He never lost hope or his faith, even in the end." Rena shared stories of him that revealed a man filled with integrity and a deep compassion for others. "He was so strong and yet so gentle and kind," she explained, reaching over to the table next to her and picking up a faded, black-and-white photo.

The picture was bent in the center from the years when it had lain folded and hidden until it could be smuggled out of Poland. Although it was faded, however, the image was clear. It showed the last vacation Rena's family ever took together, at the old farmhouse near the water where they went every summer. In the picture a strikingly handsome man stands with one arm on his hip and the other resting comfortably on the fence post outside the cabin. This is Rena's father. His hair is thick and his smile wide. He is wearing a one-piece bathing suit, typical for men at that time. The right strap is secure over his shoulder, but the left strap dangles loose across his chest. Standing next to him is Rena's mother, Rozia, wearing a bathing suit and smiling, her arms resting on Rena's shoulders. Rena is wearing a one-piece bathing suit and a wide-brimmed hat. She is about seven or eight years old. In front of them her aunt sits cross-legged on the ground, laughing.

Rena gently touched the picture. She laughed as she noticed how she had allowed one of her bathing-suit straps to dangle so that it matched her father's. "I wanted to be just like him," she said. "I loved him so much and always felt safe when he was around. I remember one year wanting to do something special for him for his birthday. I knew that one of his favorite possessions was his beautiful pocketwatch. I knew he loved that watch. The watch had a long, gold, plain chain attached to the end. Several days prior to his birthday, I asked my mother to take me to the store, where I carefully selected many shiny beads. I worked tirelessly to string them together to create a long strand to hold his watch in place alongside the chain. He carried it with him in his right pocket every day. I felt so proud. When he would hold me or hug me, I would hear that watch ticking. It made me smile. It was the sound of my Dad."

The voice of her father and the sound of his watch kept Rena's spirit alive through the starvation, the bitter cold, the torture, and the humiliation of the concentration camp, despite the horrific sights and the smell of death that floated over her head. "I would close my eyes and, in my mind, move myself from the concrete bed of the barracks and into his arms," she said. It was his voice and his message of holding on to hope and putting faith in humanity that kept her spirit alive from one moment to the next.

The Loss of Innocence

Rena's first experience of anti-Semitism occurred when she was just a child. She was in the first grade. "I remember playing outside with my friend, and another little girl walked by and threw a stone at me and called me 'a dirty Jew.' I didn't understand. I went home and asked my mother why she would say that, because I had showered and was wearing clean clothes. I was not dirty. Why would she call me that?"

"I didn't understand hate," Rena explained to me. "When you are not taught to hate, it is hard to explain or understand. I was sheltered in my little town, but I knew that in other areas anti-Semitism was strong. I understood that it was easier to be a Polish child than a Jewish child in Poland, but I was young and protected." In Poland, anti-Semitism was encouraged by the government and the church. In small towns, where many could not read or write, the townspeople often learned life lessons in the church. In many of these churches, stories were told about how the Jews had killed Christ and how Jewish people were kidnapping Polish children and using their blood to make matzo. People believed these outrageous fabrications because the stories came from sources they trusted—their churches and their leaders.

The worst time for Jews to go out in these towns was during Easter, when young students from local universities would look for Jews to harass in retaliation for Christ's death. Many believed that their problems and worries all stemmed from the Jews. They persecuted the Jews in order to make themselves feel strong and entitled by contrast. And these were the seeds of separation that Hitler treasured and promoted. We may wonder how so many could follow Hitler and his beliefs. The answer is that these messages of blame and hate were repeated so many times that they seemed to become facts, and before long it was easy for people to believe that Jews were indeed the problem and that their elimination would make life better. The daily lessons of hate paved the way for people to see Jews as less than human, which made it easier in turn to treat them with cruelty. Similar behavior today arises with bullying, blaming, and then separation, a progression that prepares the road for future violence.

At only ten years old, Rena witnessed first-hand both violence and indifference. When she was getting ready to enter the fifth grade, her mother took her shopping. It was the first time that Rena was old enough to pick out her own fabric for her school dress. She was so proud. "I examined all of the fabrics, but one caught my eye. It was white cotton, with beautiful red flowers," she said. "We bought the fabric and took it to my cousin to create my dress. I described for her the sleeves the collar and the waist that I wanted." Her cousin was a talented dress-maker. She could go to the movies, see a dress, and then go home and make it. She finished Rena's dress just before the school-year began. Rena remembers putting the dress on to wear for a family wedding that summer. "Standing there in my beautiful red-flowered dress, with my long thick braids, I felt pretty."

She couldn't know that she would never wear that dress again—that it was the last time she would ever feel pretty, or truly happy, or innocent.

In the fall of 1939, German soldiers invaded Krakow. Stories of soldiers entering other towns and killing people had already begun to spread, but

Rena's father kept telling his wife and daughter to be calm. He believed that the war would not last long because the world would hear about what was happening and come to help. They believed him—Rena believed him. But in a place deep inside, she wondered if her father might be wrong. The stirring of a fear that she had never known was beginning to rustle in the pit of her stomach.

Her fear was confirmed on a bitterly cold day when soldiers banged on their door, carrying instructions that the Ferbers were to leave their home immediately, taking only one suitcase and a pushcart. They were being relocated to the ghetto against their will because they were Jews.

Rena and her family had to pack up quickly and leave their beautiful, three-bedroom home. Rena remembers walking from room to room, looking at all of their things. "They were the things that made us a family—my mother's china, the kitchen balcony where I would call to my grandmother, and our pictures. I remember entering my room for the last time. I took in the view." On a chair sat her five porcelain Shirley Temple dolls, one with a bonnet, one holding a purse, and the others in delicate lace dresses. On her desk was her collection of Charles Dickens' novels, which her parents had bought for her as a reward for her good grades. Her new shoes, made of handpicked leather, were sitting near her bed, waiting to be worn for the first time.

Rena's voice cracked as she said, "My eye then went to my closet, where my beautiful white cotton dress with the red flowers was hanging, and I started to cry. I would not get to wear this dress to school." Then came the thought that as a ten-year-old she tried hard to wipe away along with her tears: "Maybe I will never get to wear it again."

During our interview she looked at me closely. "I think deep down I understood that we would never see our home and our things again," she said. That day, when Rena took one last look around her room and closed the door, she left the little girl in the flowered cotton dress behind. She was now an enemy of the state, in a fight for her survival. Swaddled in many layers, wearing heavy, warm boots, Rena helped her parents shove pillows, soap, extra socks, and undergarments into the suitcase.

The pushcart they filled with blankets and a big quilt. Then they began to move through the chaos in the streets to the center of town, where German soldiers were organizing the Jews' departure to the ghetto. During the process, they announced that anybody under twelve years old would not be given a permit to work in the ghetto but instead would be sent to farms to help grow food for the soldiers. Rena's parents did not want her to be separated from them, and in those frantic few minutes they managed to alter her birth certificate so that it read 1931 instead of 1929. "It was fortunate that I was tall for my age, and it was not questioned. I was now a twelve-year-old on paper, and I was granted a work permit and allowed to be sent to the ghetto with my parents."

Large trucks arrived, carrying more soldiers with guns and vicious dogs. The soldiers began separating parents from children. "People were screaming and crying, and the guards were beating and shooting them. It was so horrible. Then more trucks arrived, with more soldiers and still more dogs. The shooting and beatings continued while we waited for our permits." Rena tightened her fist as she recalled the scene.

At that time there were 40,000 Jewish people living in Krakow, but when the day was over only 25,000 had received permits to enter the ghetto; the rest were taken away in the trucks. At the time, Rena thought that the others were going to work on the farms, but now she knows that they were sent to the death camps and killed. Rena's voice grew stronger as she said, "What continues to anger me—this many years later—is the scene in the streets. While we were being killed, tortured, children ripped from parents, screaming and shooting, chaos everywhere, across the street the rest of the town carried on. The stores were open for business. Children went to school. People were moving about the streets. They didn't see us." While the rest of the town was also occupied by the Germans, only the Krakow Jews became slaves. "We were the Jews—people looked at us, but nobody saw us," Rena said.

Yet, as they left their home en route to the ghetto, Rena held onto the hope that she would someday return to their old life. Her father reassured them that the horror would not last.

She and her parents, grandparents, aunts, uncles, and cousins all arrived at the Krakow ghetto that afternoon. It was the middle of the day when they passed over the bridge and were able to see the city on the horizon. At the center of the Podgorze district, the ghetto that had once housed 3,000 people was now crowded with more than 17,000 displaced outcasts. Their eyes took in the view, but their minds struggled to comprehend what they were seeing. The city that they loved was transformed. New walls of stone had been constructed—tall walls with gates. The city had become a prison. All around them were armed guards and hundreds of dogs, trained to tear people apart for any reason or no reason—simply on command.

Once inside the gates, her father held Rena close and whispered in her ear not to be afraid because the war would not last long. She heard his words and filed them away deep inside her, where nobody could touch them. She felt safe in his embrace. She clung to his words of hope like a life-preserver. While she didn't understand it at the time, her father's words would become the very blood of her survival—the difference between allowing death and battling for life.

The Expectations of a Child

At only ten years old, Rena needed what normal children her age need: protection. She needed to be taken care of, nurtured, and made to feel safe—all the things that she had left back in her old bedroom with her flowered dress. Her new reality was a small dirty room, where a sheet hung to separate her family from the other family who shared the room. They were living on the fourth floor of a cold and damp building, with outdoor toilets and water that ran cold, if it ran at all. The water and electricity were turned on only at certain times of the day, which made staying clean and warm impossible.

The businesses that had once been owned by Rena's Jewish neighbors were now moved to the ghetto, and ownership was transferred to the Germans. Rena began to work in a print shop with her mother, while her father worked for the Jewish police. Everyone worked, but they received no wages. "We were slaves," Rena stated flatly. The family worked twelve hours a day under horrible conditions, yet they were grateful for the work because it kept them alive.

Life in the ghetto was hard. During our interview Rena looked up at me with a sad smile. "It is odd the things that you remember this many years later. We were only in the ghetto for a short while when my mother told me I had to get my hair cut short. It may seem like a small thing as I tell you. But with so many other losses, it was one more part of me—my little ten-year old-self—that was being taken away." Rena understood that in their poor living conditions, taking care of her long hair was too difficult. But after it was cut off, Rena avoided looking at herself in the mirror. Who was she becoming? She was beginning to feel as if she possessed only shattered fragments of herself. She remembers reaching up and pulling at the short locks as if she could lengthen them. "I still wanted to feel pretty. But for whom? I didn't know. Maybe for me. Perhaps my hair—my appearance—was what made me feel normal and healthy, like myself again. I longed to feel human."

With her curly, thick, dark hair lying on the floor, the little ten-year-old turned her head so that her mother wouldn't see her tears. But when she returned to their one-room home and her father saw her short hair, he began to cry. He hugged her, and they both sobbed. In his embrace, she could hear the pocketwatch tick. She felt for a moment as though they were back at home. They would be safe, and life would return—these were her private thoughts, but the aching feeling in her stomach warned her otherwise.

They lived in fear of the banging sound of soldiers at their door. They had witnessed neighbors being pulled out of their homes and dragged away. These sights and the fear of being taken to another camp dominated their thoughts. "We really did think that people were being moved around to other camps to work." Rena glanced out the window of her Florida home, and her voice dropped to a whisper. "How could we have ever imagined the truth? How could the mind have ever imagined that the Germans, such smart, cultured, educated people, could be capable of the horror that was to be revealed to us?"

On a particularly hot and sunny summer day, Rena's family learned that her grandparents would not be granted their permits to remain in the ghetto and would soon be taken away. Rena panicked. The gravity of what that meant was clear by now. If her grandparents were taken away, they would not be going to work in the fields. They would die. Stories about the death camps were beginning to circulate, and a new fear was pulsing in the air. Her family quickly moved into action. In front of the old building they were staying in was a large, overgrown courtyard, filled with piles of leaves and old, broken baskets. Rena's mother and grandparents dug a tunnel in the dirt, and her mother told Rena to hide there with her grandparents.

"My mother covered us with dirt and leaves and placed the old baskets on top of us and then rushed off to work. We lay there, holding onto the dirt without moving, for so many hours." Suddenly the ground started to shake and dogs barked. Rena was petrified. She could hear the soldiers shooting and people screaming. The dogs were barking, and the ground vibrated. She closed her eyes and tried not to move; her heart was pounding. She heard the guards running down the stairs of their building and into the courtyard. "I knew they were around us. I could feel that they were nearby. I held my breath. And then silence. And then more silence. No dogs, no guns, no footsteps."

After a short period of time had passed, Rena felt somebody moving the dirt off them. It was her mother, telling them to hurry. They stood up quickly and began to brush the dirt off. In our interview Rena smiled at me as her eyes filled with tears. "I can still feel my grandmother's hands running through my hair, wiping out the leaves and dirt." She paused, as if she were back there in Krakow, feeling that gentle touch.

But while they were running back to their building, two young guards appeared out of nowhere and asked for their papers. Her grandparents stood still. They had nothing to produce. The guards instructed them to come with them. Rena began to scream, begging them not to take her grandparents. Her screaming got louder and almost involuntary. "My voice was loud, my tears were there, but they didn't hear me. Nobody heard me. Nobody saw us." Rena's voice cracked.

As I sat still in my chair, listening to her words, I wondered how people back then could have failed to see her. How could so many have turned away and made her invisible? What kind of human beings were her neighbors and friends? And then I wondered: would it really be different today? Or is there truth to the notion that respect and tolerance are given only to those whom we believe are similar to ourselves? The "other" remains removed from us—their stories and suffering are not within our understanding and therefore do not seem to be our responsibility.

Rena's voice became soft as she said, "Sometimes, when I sleep, I can still see my grandparents walking away, holding hands. They never looked back as I was crying and screaming. My sweet grandmother, who loved me, hugged me, braided my hair, and taught me my multiplication, was being taken away. It was an unbearable pain. She was gone."

Although it had been only a week since their arrival to the ghetto, it seemed like years. Rena's grandparents were gone, and their lives were filled with constant fear. The sound of barking dogs, gunshots, and screaming never stopped. The soldiers would come banging on doors, pulling people from their homes, at any time of the day or night. It was the sound that they feared most but waited for constantly, and it came for them one late afternoon. The Gestapo arrived at their door with accusations that her father was a traitor. He was pulled from the house and arrested. Rena and her mother learned later that day that one of her father's friends had accused him of being part of the underground resistance in order to win his own freedom. Her mother was frantic to correct the error and sent Rena to the jail to beg for his release. But when Rena entered the jail, the guards would not listen to her. Rena sat on the floor and began to sob.

Then one of the guards approached her, put his hand on her shoulder, and escorted her into her father's cell to say good-bye.

Rena paused before continuing her story. "It is so funny how this many years later I can still see that guard's face," she said. "In a place filled with evil, cruel, and callous hearts, this one act of compassion gave me hope."

As she hugged her father tight, with tears running down her face, he whispered in her ear that the war would end soon and that the world would come to their rescue. Hold on to hope, he said. Her father was taken away two days later. It wasn't until many years after the war that Rena uncovered the truth about his death. She had believed that he was sent to Auschwitz and killed, but his name was not in the records. "The Germans kept very good records, as they were very proud of the number of deaths that they had recorded," she said with obvious bitterness. An eyewitness later told her that her father had been taken outside the gates of the ghetto and shot—shot by the very guard who had showed compassion to her.

It is hard to understand how the human mind can justify acts of violence sprinkled with acts of kindness. For many Nazis, killing seemed to be only a job. They did what they were told without questioning the moral issue, and so they became indifferent to killing. But with her father gone, Rena remembers, true despair began to grip her.

Hope Is the Breath of Survival

For two long years, Rena and her mother worked in the ghetto. Each day, and sometimes several times a day, the guards would invade their homes and workshops. Without any understanding of who would be taken next or why, people were removed and put into big trucks parked in the middle of the ghetto, and from there they were taken to the death camps. Those who remained in the ghetto thought that these other camps had been given the name "death camps" because the labor there was harder and the guards crueler. During our interview, Rena rubbed her hands and stared at them. "How could we have ever imagined the truth of the camps that we were being taken to? The mind can't fathom that kind of horror. Even today, having lived through it, I can't imagine it. It is no wonder that the rest of the world could not believe it—would not believe it. It remains unthinkable even today. There are still no adequate words to describe it." She stared off into the distance.

Living in the ghetto meant learning how to deal with chronic fear, unpredictable cruelty, and an uncertain but terrifying future. There was always a change coming, and it was always worse than what had happened before. What came next for Rena and her mother was a move from the ghetto to a place up the hill about seventeen kilometers to the Plaszow work camp. The move stirred a new fear in Rena—the safety of her little cousin Jenny.

Rena and her mother had been hiding the toddler in their room since the day that Jenny's mother was taken away. Now the guard gave the order for Rena to go and pack only one suitcase before reporting back to their work station. Rena turned to her mother, who whispered to her to take Jenny to the orphanage for safekeeping. Rena ran through the streets back to their tiny, shared space and opened the door. She found her little cousin Jenny sound asleep on the floor, just as they had left her earlier that morning. At only three years old, she looked utterly innocent, with bright blue eyes and curly blonde hair.

Rena let Jenny sleep as she packed the suitcase with blankets, a sheet, socks, and undergarments. She slipped on her snowsuit and heavy boots and then grabbed a small picture of her father and placed it in the bottom of the suitcase. She glanced at the pocketwatch sitting on the table, with the beaded chain she had made for him. "I knew I could not take the pocketwatch with me—valuable items were forbidden," she told me. Rena remembers looking down at the beautiful, innocent Jenny sleeping. She knew she was doing the right thing, the only thing possible. She woke the child, took one last look at the pocketwatch, then led Jenny out the door and closed it behind them. Holding her suitcase in one hand and Jenny's hand in the other, she took the little girl to the entrance of the orphanage.

As she and I spoke of this, Rena looked out the window, and the tears she had been fighting throughout her story broke loose. "I reassured

Jenny that she would like it there at the orphanage. I told her she would be able to play with other children. In my mind, I imagined the orphanages back home that were run by Catholic nuns. How could I have ever imagined that as we were leaving the ghetto they were already starting to kill the children? How could we have known? How could we have imagined? I can still hear the gunshots as they killed all the beautiful children." Rena looked at me. Her eyes were glazed with tears and dark sadness. She squeezed the tissue she was holding and said, "This haunts me still."

Hope is the very breath of survival, instilling life into the lifeless, strength into the weak, and courage into the scared. In my hometown of Cleveland, Ohio, we have witnessed first-hand the incredible strength of hope. For ten years, our local television stations covered the story of two missing girls: Amanda Berry and Gina DeJesus. When they first went missing, we watched as their pictures were posted on the screen and an active FBI search began. Then, in each year that followed, we viewed the remembrance gatherings and heard the families' pleas for the FBI to keep searching. We listened to the interviews of Amanda's mother and sister as they begged for her return. Many participated in the rallies and search parties organized by Gina's family. They never stopped looking for the girls. They never lost hope that they were alive and that they would find them. They clung to hope even as the years passed. Through the lenses of the television cameras, the two families spoke to Amanda and Gina, begging them to come home if they could and to know that they were searching for them.

What we as a community learned—ten years later—is that the girls were actually listening. On a little black-and-white TV, a few feet from the bed they were chained to, they heard and saw the hope and determination of their families, friends, and community. We learned that it was not just two girls but three, being held captive for more than ten years in the home of a deranged man, not far from their own homes. They survived torture, starvation, rape, and indescribable cruelty. They lived on hope and survived. On that miraculous day, May 6th, 2013, Michelle Knight, Amanda Berry, and Gina DeJesus escaped from their hell, and our town witnessed how hope leads to survival. During a national broadcast with Robin Roberts, these incredible young women left us all with a strong message about survival. As she looked directly into the camera, Amanda said, "Never give up on hope."

Survival. It is not simply about being alive—it is about remaining alive with endurance, perseverance, and a persistent will to outlast the trauma, the tormentors, and the guilt. Rena understood that to survive what was facing her, she would need to cling hard to hope. She held firm to the belief that she could outlast the cruelty, the humiliation, and her own survivor's guilt. Likewise, the three survivors in Ohio managed to keep their hope alive through an unthinkable ordeal. In the story of these extraordinary women, we learn that when we can find a way to nurture hope, we can discover our deepest strengths and, with that, the determination to live—and even thrive.

CHAPTER 8

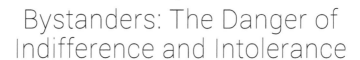

Bystanders: The Danger of Indifference and Intolerance

"The world will not be destroyed by those who do evil,
but by those who watch them without doing anything."

— ALBERT EINSTEIN

WHEN WE READ or hear stories about genocide and the Holocaust, our natural tendency is to see them as something terrible that happened in our past, in our history, but not in ourselves. After all, today we are a more enlightened and sophisticated society. We are more educated and knowledgeable, and our world is now globally connected. We see and know things in a way that people couldn't in the past.

But indifference is not a lack of knowing—it is a lack of interest in knowing. We don't want to know about the genocides today in Rwanda, Darfur, Sudan, Nigeria, and Armenia, just as we don't want to know about ongoing racism. This is not because we are uncaring but because we are disconnected. What happens somewhere else, to other people, is seemingly not part of our own existence.

Bystanders are defined as onlookers, non-participants, observers, or eyewitnesses to an event or action. Bystander apathy is a social psychological phenomenon in which witnesses refuse to help a victim, particularly if others are around. The underlying assumption is that somebody else will do something. Such apathy indicates a refusal to understand, intellectually and emotionally, the pain and suffering of others—particularly those who are different from us.

Bystanders follow the lead of those around them. If others begin a dialogue about genocide, racism, and injustice, or if they raise awareness, demonstrating emotions regarding these issue, the bystanders are more likely to become connected.

In addition, bystanders suffer from confusion about what role they can or should play, because they lack confidence in their ability to make a difference. "What can I possibly do about killings in another country?" they ask themselves. When we feel ill-equipped to make a difference, we cope by ignoring the images and facts we encounter. Bystanders see injustice and yet make a conscious choice to do nothing. It seems to me that this is how indifference, apathy, and disconnection become the seeds of hate and prejudice. Such feelings creep in like small cancer cells, undetected and seemingly benign, and we ignore them. But if they are left unchecked, they will spread and destroy what is healthy, creating an ever-growing, life-threatening tumor.

Human beings are wired for good, for compassion, and for connections, just as they are wired for survival. The Nazi guards, Rena's non-Jewish friends who closed their blinds and chose not to see her family being led away, and the people who looked out their windows and saw human hair and ashes floating in the wind—they all had to re-wire themselves. They washed their brains with thoughts that the Jews were to blame for their problems and that their own survival would be at risk if the Jews lived. They used words like "others" and "them" in order to create an emotional distance. They gave themselves permission to feel disconnected in an effort to preserve their own souls. This disconnectedness started stealthily, with laws and rules that limited the rights of Jews. Then, once these rules were intellectually accepted, it became easier for people to treat Jews differently, indeed to see them differently. What followed was a disconnection from empathy, which invited hate, terror, and violence.

Bias: Beliefs and Our Brain

Rena Finder, survivor of the Holocaust, gave me a sad smile as she said, "I wish I were telling you a story of something that occurred to me back then—but look around, it is happening now. Discrimination and intolerance exists." Racism, sexism, anti-Semitism, ageism, classism, bias, and prejudice not only exist overtly, through obvious labeling, judging, and acts of discrimination, but continue to spread insidiously in covert and unconscious ways.

We create policies, reframe history, construct rules, speak on God's behalf, train and educate each other, all through the filters of our subconscious biases. When we acknowledge these biases, however, and expose our minds to ideas and views that run counter to stereotypical messages, we can limit and control our biases and prevent the spread of hate and violence.

It takes great intellectual and emotional effort to override our stubborn biases and beliefs. In fact, research has demonstrated that the amygdala, an area of the brain associated with fear-processing and automatic thinking, is active during initial racial prejudice. Here is how it works. The amygdala is in part responsible for making connections between unpleasant experiences and our reactions or beliefs. For example, the amygdala will hold on to the connection between a particular restaurant and a food-poisoning experience that occurred there. Even if you tell yourself that it may never happen again, the association is strong, and your physiological reaction and memory of the experience will remain vivid. Consequently, your behavior will be influenced, and you will be unlikely to eat at that restaurant again. Research has demonstrated that this connection applies to our prejudices as well. One study demonstrated that participants with a strong racial prejudice had to work hard to disconnect the words "black" and "bad." This is a clear reminder of how prejudice and hate can become automatically linked in a way that makes the hate falsely appear rational and factual.

As I listened to Rena's stories about indifference and intolerance, I tried to imagine myself looking out the window and seeing my neighbors being forcibly taken away. Would I also close my blinds out of fear and self-preservation? How would I justify that behavior to myself? Would I tell myself that there really wasn't anything I could do? Or worse, would I reassure myself that what was happening out there had nothing to do with me? I'm not Jewish, gay, Muslim, or black. Can I really risk inserting myself into the lives of others to see, hear, and feel the world through their eyes? Doesn't this put me at greater risk, and shouldn't I follow my instinct to protect myself?

Bystanders aren't created spontaneously—we don't suddenly become inert to the needs of others. It happens one subtle thought at a time. It begins when we give ourselves permission to deny our own ugly biases and then draw conclusions as if our prejudices were facts. How easy it is for all of us, myself included, to ignore our biases and not face ourselves. Rena pointed out that today Germany does not have the death penalty. To justify killing, even in response to crimes, would be opening the wound, the sin of their history. In the United States, we also have a sin, a wound that we don't want to look at: slavery, and the ongoing racism that continues to breathe strong.

As a white woman, I realize that I can no longer expect my black friends to ease me into racial conversations, or take care of my feelings, or protect me from acknowledging my unintentional and covert thoughts—thoughts that, in their own way, help to keep racism alive. Rena reminded me to nurture in myself the hardest kind of courage: moral courage.

I thought about one of my dearest friends, Dr. Deborah Plummer, and wondered how many times she had danced around issues of racism with me, how often she had sugarcoated stories to protect my white feelings. I knew I owed her more than that. I owed her an honest conversation that would break the comfortable and increasingly deafening silence around me.

Racists Come in Different Shades of Kindness and Color

I first met Debbie when I was a senior in high school, when her name was still Sister Phyllis Marie. She taught me many classes, including Psychology, at Notre Dame Academy, an all-girls Catholic high school. Sister Phyllis—or simply Phyllis, as we often called her, much to the displeasure of the Mother Superior and our Principal—was our favorite teacher. We didn't much care about the consequences that followed whenever we were caught using the name; we meant it in a playful and affectionate way. No other nun had earned this kind of respect and affection from us, just Phyllis.

Our homeroom was part of the school's addition, which had been built several years before I became a student there and was always cold. It did have some advantages, however. First, it was at the end of the building and therefore removed from the rest of the school, which meant fewer supervising eyes. Second, the hallway of the addition had been built on a hill that lent itself to fun games of rolling and sliding. Finally, because of the impaired heating system, our room had an added heater, equipped with vents that blew warm air, and these gusts felt great against the bare skin that my Catholic uniform revealed. I liked to sit on that radiator every morning in homeroom.

Sister Phyllis had different ideas: she thought we should sit in our actual seats. She tried her very best to exert control over the classroom, bless her heart. She used a stern voice, made threats, and promised consequences. But we were seniors in an all-girls Catholic high school, and we were getting weary of all the rules. We knew that Sister Phyllis Marie was really just "one of us." She was not much older than we were, had a great sense of humor, liked music, and really liked to dance. So homeroom would go like this.

Sister Phyllis Marie: "Lori, get off the heater and into your seat."

"Come on Phyllis, it's freezing in here," I would sweetly say.

Cue the music, and homeroom would become a dance fest with a lot of laughing. Sister Phyllis would be in the center of it all, dancing away.

She was smart, funny, and inspirational. She was the keeper of our se-crets. She championed us and challenged us. She saw value and worth in each of us, even when we couldn't see it in ourselves. We trusted, loved, and admired her. She wasn't like the other teachers; she was more like one of us. Yes, we truly believed that she was one of us—meaning, white. But the truth was that Sister Phyllis Marie was not "one of us"—she was black. In fact, she was the only black teacher in the school and the only black nun in the Order.

As a child, Sister Phyllis was known as Debbie. She was the daughter of a Jamaican mother and an African-American father and experienced discrimination from a young age. As a little girl entering middle school in the 1960s, Debbie saw hate, and it scared her. She remembers the story of her godparents hitting the front page of the local newspaper in Cleveland. They had become victims of hate crimes when they tried to move into a predominantly white neighborhood. After observing these crimes and seeing the tension and fear in the city and local suburbs, Debbie's parents made the decision to move their family out of the city into a small, remote, rural town. They bought property and built a home. The family was excited as they watched their new home take shape. But not everyone shared their joy.

One day, as Debbie and her family drove down the street in their new hometown, they were greeted by the sight of barbed wire. Their next-door neighbor had put up a tall fence with "No Trespassing" signs placed along the perimeter. This welcome-wagon committee suggested that perhaps Debbie and her family should go and live with "their own kind." When it became clear that Debbie's family would not be intimidat-ed by the fence or by signs and hurtful words, the neighbor replaced his American flag with a Confederate flag. The flapping of the flag was vis-ible from Debbie's bedroom window. It served as a daily reminder and a clear message: she was not welcome because her skin was black. Anxiety and fear stirred in her each morning when she saw that potent symbol of hate.

Debbie's sisters coped with the racism by fighting back. "They would say, 'If they're so afraid of me I'll act even scarier,'" she told me many years later. Her siblings rebelled and became angry. Debbie took a different approach, reminding herself daily to "be polite, be clean, be friendly, be smart, be funny. Make them like me. Then maybe they will like other black people as well." Even as a young girl, she took on the tremendous responsibility of changing how white people viewed her and, by extension, how they viewed all black people. It was her mission: Prove them wrong. Let them see that I am just like them. She remained vigilant, trying always to be good and to ingratiate herself to white people. But this vigilance kept fear and anxiety alive at her core.

Debbie's mother showed her how to push through what she generously called "ignorance" in their neighbors. She reassured Debbie, "They are just ignorant and scared—once they get to know us, it will be different. Once they see that we won't be spitting watermelon seeds and putting a grill on the porch and barbecuing every night, they will accept us." Debbie's family laughed as her mother said this. She maintained her cheery disposition and continued to wave and greet their neighbors every day, despite their constant hurtful words and actions.

Because their neighbors' racism was overt and intentional, Debbie could see it and navigate around it, even though it was painful. She became used to being the "other" and the "only" in high school, and again when she entered the convent. But an even greater struggle arrived for Debbie when she had to deal with the subtle and at times unconscious racism of those who believed they weren't prejudiced.

Debbie worked diligently to be a black role model. She was quick to add, "All of my teachers, superiors in the convent, and executive bosses up to the present have all been white." But she carries residual anxiety with her to this day. "It is as if I am still working to never give anybody a reason to put up a barbed-wire fence, or judge me simply because I am black," she said. "So I overcompensate by never being late, by being polite, neat, and organized." She also never spits watermelon seeds.

When Intolerance and Religion Intersect

When Sister Phyllis Marie entered the convent, she had a clear expectation of how she would be received. The convent would be a non-judgmental place of acceptance, she thought, a place that would remove obstacles from her spiritual life in order for her to get closer to God. That was where Sister Phyllis Marie longed to be—in a place where everyone was equal in God's eyes, and where acceptance would be deeply felt by all, including her; a place where she would not have to work so hard to be accepted as her true self.

What she actually found in her convent life were yet more obstacles. It turned out that just because her fellow nuns believed in God, read Scripture, and followed the rules of the Order, they were not less judging, less intolerant, or less biased.

When I spoke to her about this time in her life, Debbie thought for a moment and then said, "I never really named it until now, but it was racism." It was visibly difficult for Debbie to reflect on her real reasons for leaving her life as a nun. This time she didn't share with me the softer, sanitized version of the story that she has told and written about before. Instead, she told the story as it really happened: she was compelled to leave the convent because of racism.

Several incidents prompted her to leave. The first occurred because in the convent she felt isolated from her culture and from parts of her identity, and she wanted other black Catholic students to have what she hadn't known: a supportive community, a place for networking and connection, a place of belonging. With guidance and support from the Catholic diocese, she started a youth group for black Catholic students in the area. It started out as a small gathering of fourteen students but soon grew to over four hundred students. Some of her fellow nuns supported her efforts and volunteered to chaperone and help with fundraising events.

The group's dances and events were held at one of the local Catholic high schools. It was the largest school in the area and could best accommodate the students. Just before one of their scheduled events, she was asked to come to a meeting at the school. She grimaced at the recollection. "There they all sat. My fellow nuns who were my friends, leaders, and administrators." Within the first few minutes, she realized that this group had met before, without her, and that the topic they were raising had been rehearsed. The conversation began with an acknowledgment that the youth group was a great "community service" and that they were happy she had "taken up the cause."

But now there was a concern, one of the Sisters explained. A parent had called and expressed concerns about all the black kids she had seen coming out of Regina High School. "The parent is beginning to reconsider sending her daughter to the high school in the fall. She is afraid that with the black youth group being hosted at the school, it's getting a black image," the Sister told Debbie. Then she added, "I didn't know what to say to her. I think we will need to look for a new location for the meetings."

Even now, repeating the Sister's words from many years ago, Debbie's reaction is one of disbelief mixed with anger. She let out a sarcastic laugh as she recounted her response. "I am really sorry that you didn't know what to say to them," she told the Sister. "I am sure there is a lot in Scripture that you could have found to guide you." She felt ambushed and betrayed by her "friends," these white nuns who clearly agreed that "a black image" was not a good one. In that moment, a deep realization hit her: her white friends, superiors, and leaders had decided that instead of working on changing the beliefs and fears of the white parents, it was better—easier—to hide the black kids. To ignore the racial prejudice that was clear and visible in the parents' comments. But when she spoke with me, Debbie added, "I understand that they didn't want to label it as racism because even I found other, softer words to describe what was happening."

The incident changed her, forcing her to look for the first time at how her own black identity fit in with this white community, which was supposedly dedicated to loving and embracing all of mankind.

Shortly after the youth-group incident, she took a group of high-school students on their annual trip to Washington, DC. This was a trip she had chaperoned many times. Public, private, and parochial schools from all over America participated in this national program. The program coordinator created room assignments and mixed up the students from different schools as part of the learning experience.

The girls were given room keys and assignments, and Sister Phyllis Marie settled into her room to prepare their schedule for the next day. Soon six girls from Notre Dame appeared in her doorway. One of them said, "You have to do something. Tina has been assigned to a room with that girl from Mississippi. You know, the black girl. She is going to have to sleep in a room with her. You know, share a room and a bathroom with the black girl." Debbie's voice took on a high pitch as she imitated the student for me.

"I just stood there, shocked," she told me. "Shocked that they felt that way and even more shocked that they were saying it to me." She chuckled as she continued the story.

Another student, who was more self-aware and sensitive, chimed in: "Oh, Sister Phyllis, this is not about you. I mean, you're not really black. We don't even consider you black."

In that moment, Debbie thought about a similar incident that had happened before they left on the trip. While she sat in her classroom grading papers, a small group of students sat on the floor with the intention of studying, though mostly they were chatting and laughing. In the midst of the laughter, she overheard one of the students playfully call the other one a "nigger." The other student put her finger to her lips and pointed toward Sister Phyllis Marie. And the first student said, "Oh, that's just Phyllis. She's not really black. You know, we like her."

Things were becoming painfully clear to Debbie. All this time, she had been putting her best self out there—her best behavior, her truest and kindest intentions. She said, "Here I thought, all this time, I was the model to show them that all black people are really no better or worse than white people. But I realized what they were doing was eliminating me from the black equation. I wasn't black to them. They liked me, respected me, and valued me because they saw me as white."

After the trip to Washington, DC, it became obvious to Debbie that she needed to leave the convent and her all-white community. She needed to reconnect with her black identity to explore her own racial views, including her own racism.

The Face of a Bystander

Of all the "isms," racism is the most emotionally charged and the hardest for Americans to discuss. More people are willing to admit to sexist views, bias around ageism, and even anti-Semitic thoughts. But mention the word "racism," and anger, defensiveness, and silence quickly follow. Yet, although it is a painful process, we must all look deeply into our conscious and unconscious biases. Until we do so, we will never be able to fully connect with each other. We will have learned nothing from stories like Rena's and Debbie's. So it is time. No more being a bystander. Let me begin the conversation.

I am white. I am a psychologist. I am an advocate. I have spent the better part of my professional career of thirty years helping and serving others—particularly those who haven't found their voices. I have several black friends. In fact one of my most cherished friends, colleagues, and mentors is a black woman. Surely that must mean I am not a racist?

In my conscious thoughts and actions, I work diligently to challenge my biases and my assumptions when they come into my awareness. How, then, can I be a racist? After all, racists are people filled with hate and entitlement, who are capable of horrible acts of violence against others. Racists are not pretty or smart or inspirational. Racists are ugly. Being a racist is a horrible and socially unacceptable thing. It is no wonder that nobody wants to step up to the microphone and say, "I am a racist."

But what if we all looked deeply into the mirror and acknowledged that we are filled with biases and beliefs and, yes, racial prejudice, which operates in the most dangerous way because it is hidden and subconscious? What if really good people, with good intentions, stepped up to the microphone and acknowledged that racism exists? Not "out there" but "in here," in all of us. In the seemingly subtle jokes, innuendo, and thoughts about marginalizing others, which we all engage in at one time or another. It exists in our words, our choices, our votes, and our behavior.

What if we as a society stopped dancing around the ugly wound that we refuse to acknowledge because it hurts too much? What if smart, kind-hearted, and well-intentioned people stepped forward and started a conversation about racism? A conversation about real tolerance—tolerance that we put into action, not the kind that makes for a great quote, Facebook message, or political slogan. No, I mean the kind that is hard, the kind that hurts, that kind that forces us to step outside of our comfort zone and imagine ourselves in the life of somebody else—somebody who looks, worships, and lives differently from us. And then, what if we accepted those people as equals, rather than just tolerating them? Perhaps then we would be able to see clearly the invisible line that is called indifference, so that we might avoid it.

Indifference: The Invisible Line between Good and Evil

When Rena Finder, a twelve-year-old girl in a concentration camp, first entered the storeroom of the death camp, she tried to take in what she was seeing. Her eyes moved around the large warehouse. It was filled with enormous piles from floor to ceiling: jewelry, clothes, dolls, suitcases, blankets, pillows, books, and shoes—so many shoes. They were the last personal belongings of the Jews who had been taken away. This was one of the hardest tasks assigned to her and her mother: they were instructed to sort the items and pack them up in boxes.

Rena stirred in her seat as she spoke to me and said, "It was emotionally hard to be touching the things of people that I knew were probably dead. Things that once defined them, that were once part of their lives." As she and her mother dug through the piles, they found fancy women's shoes with beautiful trim, men's work shoes, baby booties, and little shoes for toddlers. "I tried to imagine the people who wore these shoes. Did the women feel pretty when they put on the fancy shoes? Did they dance in them? Were the little shoes the ones that the babies took their first steps in? Did the baby doll bring comfort and joy to a little girl? Did she cry when it was taken from her? I thought about my things: my father's watch, my dolls, my books, and of course my beautiful white dress with red flowers. Where were those items? Was somebody touching, packing, or wearing my things—my dress and new shoes?"

Her voice trailed off. Then she became irritated. "Can you believe it was our job to sort through these items? And then, worse, we had to package them to be shipped to the home of German soldiers." It seems inconceivable, but the ugly reality was that soldiers' families wore the clothes of people they had killed. Their children played with the dolls of babies whose lives they had taken. Their wives danced in the shoes of women they had tortured. It is almost impossible to comprehend emotionally what they were doing. How could they disconnect themselves in that way?

Rena reached over to the table, lifted a glass of water, and slowly took a sip. As she placed the glass back on the table, I saw that her hands were trembling. She crossed her legs at the ankles. It was the first time, over the last several hours, that she had moved in her chair. She looked at me, shook her head, and sighed. "Indifference—we were seen as something, somebody, separate, and different from them, less than. That's how they did what they did."

Rena was right. Indifference, disconnection, and lack of compassion for others set the stage for millions of human beings to become invisible, unseen—for the people around them to stand by and emotionally disconnect themselves from the "others." Indifference allowed a man to offer a cup of coffee to a friend, hug and kiss his family, pray to God, and then place his fellow human beings into ovens to burn. The brightest minds of Germany were building gas chambers, while their devout religious leaders preached about "us" and "them," facilitating a separation and encouraging indifference and intolerance. Seemingly good people were shopping and sending their children off to school while within their vision other children were being shot.

It was the invisible and silent line between good and bad, right and wrong, human and inhuman, that allowed this behavior to happen. This line of indifference can creep into our souls when we are not paying attention and override our natural instinct to help.

We are born with a sensitivity and an awareness of the needs of others. Children as young as six months old prefer images of people helping others, and toddlers are often eager to "make it better" when they see somebody crying. Our challenge is to pay attention to that innate desire and to find the courage to acknowledge our quiet and often hidden thoughts of indifference. The choice to get involved and engage can often be complicated by concerns for our own safety, fears of how we will be perceived by others, beliefs that somebody else will step in, and our personal relationship with the person in need. But when I look at our history and our daily news, I continue to see that in every tragic event, there are many who instinctively run to help. Where there is hate and bullying, I hear many morally courageous people speaking out. Standing by silently as others suffer is not in our nature; it is a behavior that we create when we refuse to step into the shoes of others. And it is a behavior we can fight to change.

CHAPTER 9

—— ❧ ——

An Upstander: Standing Up for Others

"May your choices reflect your hopes, not your fears."

— Nelson Mandela

Sitting on his horse on a mountainside, a man dressed in an expensive suit and crisp shirt, with a gold swastika pin attached to his jacket lapel, stares at the town below. On a second horse next to him a beautiful woman, with dark, thick hair pulled back in a neat clip, moves back and forth in her saddle—restless. The two look down at the town of Krakow, Poland. The scene below contains chaos and terror: Nazi soldiers dragging people out of their homes, taking their belongs and throwing them in the streets, lining Jews up against the buildings and shooting them, dragging children from parents. One little girl in a red coat wanders the streets unseen.

The man on the horse cannot take his eyes off of the scene, barely blinking, his eyes transfixed. He watches as men, women, and children are brutalized and killed. His companion turns her head away and pulls on the reins of her horse. Her voice trembling, she begs for them to leave. The man remains still; he continues to stare at the horrors below.

For most of us, this is our first introduction to the man named Oskar Schindler. The scene is from Steven Spielberg's 1993 movie, "Schindler's List." According to Spielberg, the movie was filmed in black and white—drained of color—to mimic the way in which the Holocaust drained life. The only color that remains is the red coat of the little girl. In this scene, Schindler wonders why nobody sees the little girl as she roams the streets.

Symbolically, she represents the global indifference that existed at that time. Individuals and governments, including that of the United States, knew of the atrocities but didn't want to acknowledge them, despite the fact that they were as visible and vivid as the little girl in the red coat.

Oskar Schindler was an ethnic German who grew up in Zwittau, a region of Czechoslovakia. In his town he was referred to as "Gauner," which means swindler. In fact, he was a gambler and a charmer who profited from the war. Far from being a good husband he was a womanizer who often had several mistresses at the same time. In 1939, he purchased an enamelware factory that had been confiscated from its Jewish owners. The factory was very successful, for it manufactured pots and pans used by the soldiers and also supplied munitions for the troops. Though Schindler made a lot of money before and during the war, he was not a great businessman; ultimately he went bankrupt—many of his businesses failed both before and after the war.

However, at some point in his journey, Schindler lost the ability to remain indifferent. The invisible line between right and wrong, good and evil, became starkly visible to him: brilliant and bright, like the little girl in the red coat. His moral conscience lost the ability to un-see what he had seen when he looked down at the liquidation of the Krakow ghetto. Instead, he actually saw the horror. Rena said, "He saw it with his eyes and his heart." He didn't wait to find out what others would do. He didn't deny what he heard and saw, as others near the camp had done. He didn't tell himself that there was nothing he could do. Rather than standing by and watching what was happening from behind a curtain, he acted.

In other words, Schindler changed. He may not have been a good man by typical moral standards, but he was not a Bystander either. Instead, he found his moral courage and became an Upstander.

The Courage to Stand Up

An Upstander is a person who makes a conscious choice to speak up and fight hate and injustice. In contrast to a bystander, who sees injustice but chooses to do nothing, an Upstander not only sees it but takes action to change it. He or she is a person who finds the courage to risk stepping emotionally and intellectually into the shoes of another, to protect and support. Upstanders are eyewitnesses to pain, suffering, and injustice, and they seize even the smallest opportunities to make a difference. When Rena and her mother entered the camp, it was the instinctive kindness of an Upstander that saved their lives.

It was March 13th, 1943, when Rena and her mother arrived at the Plaszow work camp, run by Amon Goeth. Though he looked human, Goeth was devoid of humanity. "He was sadistic and cruel," Rena said. "The evil that was Amon Goeth could not be imagined." She crossed her arms and shivered. "He would kill for reasons that could not be predicted. He would at times wake up and sit on his balcony and shoot people as they worked below. Or command his attack dogs to tear people apart. He seemed to enjoy the blood and torture. People could not rest. They could only live in fear every moment." For the year that Rena was in the camp, she recalled that she never directly looked at this man. "I would move my eyes above or below. I convinced myself that if I didn't see him, then he wouldn't see me, and then maybe I would be safe."

Life in the camp was much worse than life in the ghetto. There was even less food, and the prisoners suffered daily cruelties under cold and inhumane conditions. They slept on shelves or on a floor, with death all around them. There were hangings and torture everywhere they looked. Rena tried not to look at all. "It was hard to see what human beings were doing to other human beings. I was losing hope," she said.

In the midst of this, stories began to circulate about a factory called Emalia, run by Oskar Schindler. He was said to be kind to his workers. Rena's mother learned that a friend of her father's was in charge of making the list for people to work in Schindler's factory. They went to him, and he agreed to place them on the list.

They soon became "Schindlerjuden"—Schindler Jews. Rena smiled at me. "Because of Oskar Schindler, I have a life. I was able to celebrate my seventeenth birthday, to get married to my husband, David, and

142

to live with him for sixty-six years. I was able to have three children, six grandchildren, and two great-grandchildren. I will be able to celebrate my eighty-seventh birthday in just a few days. Because one man stood up and pushed past the indifference and apathy that was all around him and within himself, I have a life."

The Life-Saving List

"At first we didn't trust Schindler because he was friends with the vile Amon Goeth and he wore a gold and diamond swastika pin," Rena explained. But over time they saw how he used his charm, his relationships with other Germans, and his ability to swindle and bribe for the purpose of keeping his workers safe. He would allow them to hold religious celebrations in the factory and would pay off guards for their silence. The workers were loyal to Schindler because he showed compassion, which they seldom saw or felt in the hell they were living in.

"If there was God, then I believed that he sent Oskar Schindler. He was like an angel. I often say that I really expected sometimes to see wings coming out of his back," Rena told me. "The day we left to work for him I felt was the true liberation for me. We went from hell to heaven. He protected us and treated us as if we were human again. He looked at us and saw us. In the midst of all of the hate and misery, Oscar Schindler showed compassion."

Schindler found medicine on the black market for Rena's diabetic friend and glasses for those who needed them. He was clever and hid his kind acts from the soldiers who frequently came into the factory. For example, he would light cigarettes and then put them down near the work stations as if he had forgotten them—a way of giving the men cigarettes. He once yelled at Rena and threw a sandwich at her. The gesture was supposed to show his anger, but the truth was that he was feeding her. He had a small clinic that offered real medical care in the factory.

On several occasions, when Amon Goeth was there, Schindler would intervene and slap his workers to give the impression that he was in control of them, but really in order to prevent Amon from stepping in and killing them.

He used his skills as a charmer, gambler, and womanizer to gather information and protect them. Rena recalled a time in the factory when an SS guard grabbed her and put a gun to her head after she had broken a machine that made bullet casings. She was crying as Schindler ran up to the guard and screamed at him, calling him an idiot for thinking that a little girl could break that big machine. "He was a human being who protected us," she said.

When word came that the Germans wanted to liquidate the camps and the factories, Schindler quickly worked out a deal to move his factory to his home in Brinnlitz, Czechoslovakia. He convinced his superiors that his plant and his workers were vital to the war effort. While the factory was being moved, the female workers would be temporarily relocated back to different camps, working in the warehouses and sorting personal items that had once belonged to Jews. Rena was not worried as they prepared for this temporary move—she knew they would be back in Schindler's plant soon.

Before they were transported, a Jewish doctor was brought in to Schindler's factory to apply tattoos to their arms. "He was a gentle man who had never done this before," Rena said. The doctor used a light touch and did not go very deep into her skin. In light ink he tattooed the letters "KL" on Rena's forearm—an abbreviation for the word "Konzentrationslager," which means concentration camp.

Rena looked down and rubbed the small red patch on her arm that is still visible. Her voice cracked as she said, "The tattoo only lasted for about two years. Every day I would rub it with dirt and sand until I was able to get it off. It was not like the tattoos that the women in Auschwitz received. Their tattoos were deep, and the ink was permanent. They took their numbered arms to their graves." Rena continued to rub the red patch and stared out the window.

L. = list number, Ln. = line number, Rel. = religion, Natn. = nationality, H. No = prisoner number,
1 42 Ju. Po. 76244 FERBER Rena 24.2.28 Metallarbeiterin
1 43 Ju. Po. 76245 FERBER Rosa 14.9.05 Metal Worker

On letterhead from his enamelware factory in Krakow, Schindler created a list of the names of the Jews who were being sent back to the Plaszow concentration camp. He added fictitious jobs in an effort to convince the SS guards that those on the list were critical to the war effort and should live. Rena's name, along with that of her mother, Rosa, appears on the original list of 1,200 Jews that Schindler identified as "critical to the war effort." Through his charm, bribery, and money he was persuasive, and these Jews survived the war.

Three hundred women with "KL" tattooed on their arms now sat waiting to be sent back to Praszow until the new Schindler factory in Brinnlitz was ready. Rena was among them. When they arrived back at the camp, she was struck by how different it seemed—vacant, with an eerie and heavy silence. What Rena and the others did not know was that, months before, everyone from the camp had been sent to Auschwitz. The Plaszow camp was to be liquidated—destroyed by having everything removed and every inhabitant killed. At the time, however, all Rena and the other women knew was that their time back at the camp was to be short and temporary. They were simply being held there while the barracks for women were constructed at Schindler's Brinnlitz plant. This realization kept their hope alive and made the tasks in the camp tolerable.

Standing Up: Choosing to Know the Horror behind the Black Iron Gate

As I sat listening to Rena and bracing myself for what was to come next, I wondered if anybody would really want to hear her story. I myself battled with the familiar argument: these stories are horrifying, appalling, and painful, so why keep retelling them? But as I listened to the most painful moments of Rena's story, I realized the truth. The horror of the concentration camps was allowed to happen because many did not want to know, see, or hear the truth. The retelling of these stories forces us all to look into the painful mirror of history and see ourselves. They remind us that we are all able to offer both harm and life-sustaining acts of kindness;

to be Upstanders and to find the courage to stand up. And the road to standing up for others begins with the first, small step of hearing and knowing painful truths.

The elderly woman sitting in front of me had found her courage to share these truths with all of us. Rena took a deep breath, stared at her hands folded in her lap, and began to retrace her journey into hell.

The two boxcars waited on the tracks like ominous black caves. But Rena and her mother thought they were simply one more thing they had to endure on their way to Schindler's plant and safety. Approximately 150 women were shoved into each of the cars. They were pushed and crammed into the boxes and forced to sit, lie, and stand on top of each other. As the doors were slammed and locked behind them, the heat hit Rena's face. She felt as if she were suffocating there in the dark, without windows, water, bathrooms, or sufficient air. All that was around her was darkness, whimpering bodies, and empty time.

It took more than a day for the train to make its way to its final destination. Rena forced her mind to focus on her father's words: "Hold on to hope—the world will save us." There in the darkness, with her legs cramping from the weight of the bodies pushing on her, filled with weakness, thirst, and hunger, Rena clung to hope. She was going to hide at Schindler's factory until the terror was over. They would be all right. Lying in the dark, hot, human pile, Rena thought she heard her father's pocketwatch ticking. She drifted off to a restless sleep.

Rena was jolted awake as the train shuddered to an abrupt stop. "We are finally here," she remembers thinking. She heard somebody outside the boxcar opening the door. At first everything seemed dark; it was near midnight, and the sky was very black. Then—as quickly and unexpectedly as a bolt of lightning—a bright spotlight hit the side of the train near the door.

Rena closed her eyes and described the image: "The first thing I saw was the barbed wire. Miles and miles of barbed wire. My stomach tightened—something was terribly wrong. And then I saw it. The sixteen-foot-long, ninety-pound, black iron sign that read '**Arbeit Macht**

Frei,' which means 'Work will make you free.'" They were at the entrance gate to Auschwitz. Because of a clerical error, the train had been sent to Auschwitz instead of Brinnlitz.

Hundreds of guards with rifles and large dogs were yelling for the prisoners to get off the train. Rena recalled the stench in the air. "It was like nothing I had ever smelled before. When I got down from the boxcar I could see white flakes in the air that looked like snow. It was so difficult to breath in the boxcar, and the air outside was so thick and crushing. I tried to reach out to catch the snow, to try and quench my thirst. But when I put my hand out a new horror hit me: the flakes were not snow. These were ashes. It was ashes all around us. It was ashes."

Tears formed in her eyes, and her voice became low. She began to whisper, as if what she was going to tell me was too excruciatingly painful and shameful to say aloud, and she glanced at me with concern, unsure whether or not I could handle what was to be revealed. Then she lowered her head and continued.

Noise. Chaos. The guards yelled for them to run and whipped them into lines. They ran, and the guards beat them, and the dogs barked. More chaos. They ran until they came to a big building—a barrack. German officers were everywhere, but at the entrance of this building stood a man in a white doctor's coat, carrying a whip. He glared at them as they approached. One by one they stood before him, and he looked them up and down with his dark eyes. As each person approached, he would yell out "Left!" or "Right!" and the person would move into the line he indicated. Rena whispered to me, "Terror began to spread to all of us as we stood there, watching and waiting our turn. What was happening? How was he choosing left versus right, and what did it mean?"

Rena soon realized that the people going to the left were older and appeared to be ill and weak. She pinched her cheeks to make them rosy and nudged the girl next to her so that she would do the same. Rena and her mother stood tall and tried to appear strong and healthy as they approached the guard in the white coat. Doctor Death stared at Rena, her mother, and her friend. He yelled out, "Right." They were saved in this first round of selection—but saved for what?

The line to the left was taken into one room, and Rena and those in her line were pushed into a different room. Rena's heart raced as they were told to strip completely and throw their clothes into a pile. From the time Rena had left the ghetto, she had carried a picture of her father in her shoe. Now, as she slipped off her shoes, the picture became visible. She did not want the guards to take it from her, so she put it in her mouth to try to hide it. But the guards were checking everyone's mouths, so Rena slipped the picture back into her shoe and thought, "I will get it when we put our shoes back on." As quickly as that thought came, it was replaced with another. Something in the air was wrong. Horror set in for the little girl, who had already been through so much. Could there be more? Rena realized in that moment, "I don't think I am ever going to see my clothes again."

The prisoners stood there, huddled naked together, in several lines. The guards were telling them not to be afraid, that they were simply going into the showers. Those were the words they used, but their faces and cruel behavior suggested something far worse. The female guards were vulgar to them as they stood there naked and vulnerable. As she told me this part of the story, Rena dropped her eyes, rubbed her hands, and whispered, "They were horrible women—the things they did to us— cruel, for their own enjoyment."

The guards shaved their hair, not with razors but with scissors. They pulled their hair and cut it brutally, taking skin and leaving the prisoners bleeding. When they had finished shaving each prisoner's head, they continued to the underarms and then the pubic area. As the prisoners stood there, bleeding and humiliated, the guards dumped a powder on their open sores to prevent lice. "It was a nightmare—a horror. I can still smell the air," Rena mumbled to me, her eyes closed. My heart began to race as I watched her. I fought tears and a rising nausea.

Rena and the others were then shoved like a herd of animals into another room. The guards kept telling them not to be scared because

148

it was not a gas chamber. Rena remembers that the words punched her hard, knocking the wind out of her: gas chamber. They had been hearing rumors from people who had escaped that such chambers existed, but they could not comprehend it. It was unthinkable. Now here she was, standing naked, shaved, and bleeding, being moved into a room they were calling a shower. Rena shuddered as she relived the memory of the women huddling together, filled with terror. Pipes covered the walls, and the ceiling was filled with rows and rows of showerheads. Rena recalled the smile on the guard's face as she shut the doors and locked them. The sound echoed through the air that was now trapped in the room with them.

The lights went out. Rena remembers such raw fear that she couldn't even cry—she was paralyzed. "I don't remember screaming or hearing screaming at that moment. Maybe I was screaming, but there were no sounds—just terror. Then the lights came back on, and we waited in horror for what would happen. Then cold water began to come down on us. It was water! It was not gas. It was water." Rena stared into space as if she were seeing it all again.

I tried hard to hold back my tears, but they ran down my face. I sat motionless in the chair across from her. I wanted to comfort her in some way, to say something or do something. But Rena didn't seem to be in the room with me any longer. She was back there, huddled naked and wet, and filled with a terror that my mind had no frame of reference to comprehend. So I sat still as the tears ran down my face.

Rena continued to look down at her hands. Then at last she took a deep breath and continued her story.

"When the water was turned off, I looked at my mother, my friends, and people I had known all my life—standing there naked, with no hair, bleeding, with eyes that were empty. They did not look the same. They were not recognizable. I started to cry as I stood there naked and wet with all the other women, and I said to mother, 'We are dead. This is death.'" Rena seemed to have sunk deeper into her chair, but her eyes never left her hands. The living room was still. Rena looked up at me, then past me, and her gaze went to the window over my shoulder. The silence hung over us.

Their wet and bleeding bodies were pushed into another room—a very cold room. They stood shivering as the guards pushed them and yelled for each of them to grab clothes and a pair of wooden Dutch shoes that were sitting out on a bench. The clothes were damp and piled on top of each other. Rena ran to a pile of wet clothes; her eye was drawn to something white sticking out. It was a dress that reminded her of the one she had left behind—her white dress with the red flowers. Rena smiled sadly as she looked up at me. "It is funny: some survivors say we wore uniforms, but I don't remember wearing a uniform. Maybe I blocked that out, and we did wear the striped uniforms. But in my mind I remember grabbing a dress from the pile—it was white, and at least in my mind it had red flowers." The dress, however, had been made for a woman four times Rena's size. "It obviously came from a woman who arrived at this place—this hell—not understanding that she would not need to look pretty. She was going to die." Rena remembers wrapping the dress around herself several times so that she wouldn't trip and then stepping into tattered Dutch shoes.

From the showers the prisoners were moved outside into a line, waiting to move into their barracks. "I remember looking around at Auschwitz," Rena said. "On one side of the road there were people walking around, but they were corpses. Their bones could be seen. They had no hair, and their eyes were looking at us but they were not in there. It was hard to look at them. I said again to my mother, 'This is hell. We have died.' I couldn't even cry. I was numb. A part of me did die that day."

When they started to move toward their barracks, Rena saw a line of people who had just entered Auschwitz from the train. "The women were wearing nice clothes, beautiful shoes, and pushing carriages with babies. The men carried suitcases and wore their hats. They did not understand that when they got on that train they were going to a place to be killed. Their beautiful shoes would go into a pile. Their belongings would be given to the German soldiers' families back home, and soon their hair would float in the air along with their ashes. We were dead, and this was hell."

The barracks were dark and damp, with shelves on the walls where people lay on top of each other. They understood now that they were simply waiting for death. The days were gray and intolerable, and yet they survived, one day after another. Rena said, "I felt my energy leaving me, my mind often numb, without a thought, just empty. I wondered if I was losing my sanity. Were the things around me real? How long would it take before death would come?"

Upstanders Existed Even in Hell

"It is odd, the things that you remember this many years later," Rena added. At Auschwitz, as in the other camps, there was a roll call each morning and evening. Rena remembers that on one particular day, when they had just been dismissed from the line, a female guard walked past the girl standing in front of Rena and slapped her across the face for talking. The girl fell to the ground, bleeding. But she had not been talking.

In that moment, Rena's mind felt clear. For the first time she was filled with anger—or no, rage. "I thought to myself, 'They are taking my things, my hair, my sanity, and I am going to die here, but they are not going to take my soul,'" she told me.

Standing tall next to the fallen girl, Rena said to the guard, "She didn't say anything!"

The guard whirled around, thrust her face close to Rena's, and screamed, "What did you say?"

Rena repeated herself. The guard hit her several times and dragged her into the barracks. There she instructed Rena to kneel on the stone pile near the chimney until she apologized.

During our interview Rena told me, "I would not apologize. She could kill me. Death was coming anyway. I wanted to die with my conscience [clear, knowing] that I didn't stand by and do nothing. " Though she had no power and was risking her own life, Rena could no longer be a silent witness to the pain and cruelty around her. She knelt there on the broken glass and stones all day, until it was time for the evening roll call, when another guard told her to get up and stand in line. The guard knew that if Rena was not in line and the number count was incorrect, not only would Rena be shot but the guard as well.

After that, Rena told me, "I was no longer willing to be a bystander to the torture and torment of others. The silence inside was taking my soul."

Another time during the roll call, two soldiers approached Rena and a friend who was standing next to her. They took the two girls out of line and across the street. Rena recalled that her mother became hysterical— screaming and crying. They all understood that being taken from the line meant torture and death. The guards shoved the girls into the barrack, which looked like a cottage. Quickly a nurse in a white uniform and hat stepped between Rena and the guard. The nurse was gentle. She stroked Rena's arm and said that she was not going to hurt the girls. "She looked at my face and smiled," Rena said. "That may seem like a very small thing, but I was starving for kindness."

Rena looked around the cottage, at the two beds with white sheets and white pillows. The room offered a clean and fresh comfort that she had not seen in years. The nurse explained that she was going to take some blood "to experiment to see if it would save a German soldier."

"I didn't understand then that it was for a blood transfusion. But what I did understand in that moment was the irony of what she was saying. She wanted the blood that ran through my veins—the veins of a dirty Jew that was no better than a rat—to be used in the body of a German to save his life."

The Voice of Upstanders

Last year I was asked to give a talk to a group of female leaders on the power of gratitude in the workplace. During our lunch break, I overheard the conversation of a group of women at the table next to mine. Their talk was filled with laughter and friendly banter, and it was obvious that they knew one another and were the senior leaders of their organization. Their conversation focused on their collective disgust with a woman named Becky, a fellow leader in their organization, who had been missing a lot of work and was late on many deadlines. One woman commented that she felt their President was overlooking Becky's absences because, well, you know, "she is the favorite, the pretty one." Another woman chimed in with the snide comment that "Maybe if I wore short skirts I could get special treatment too." They all laughed and continued to discuss Becky's wardrobe, weight, and "little southern accent." I glanced over at the group, who were clearly enjoying their "bonding experience."

One of the women noticed my glance and told me how much she was enjoying my talk. She took a sip of water and added, "I really like the concept of using gratitude to build morale in our teams to increase our productivity. I am looking forward to hearing more this afternoon." Then she returned to her table's discussion of Becky. There was more talk, filled with words like "lazy" and "entitled."

A few minutes later, I heard it: the quiet, timid voice of one of the junior members of the team. She cleared her throat and said, "This conversation is making me very uncomfortable. I don't think that many of you know Becky at all, and yet you are talking about her as if you do." The young woman stood up. "I am embarrassed to sit here with you," she said, and she moved to another table. I could see that she was shaking.

The women at the table sat still for a moment and then began to express their outrage at the "disrespectful" way that their junior colleague had treated them. One woman in a beautiful suit commented that perhaps the young lady needed to learn a thing or two about gratitude and respect, if she was going to continue to work in their organization.

After the lunch break, I went to the podium again. But instead of opening up my slides, I began with a story. I introduced the concept of being an Upstander and the courage it takes to stand up for someone else, to correct an injustice rather than passively participating in belittling banter for the sake of fitting in. I stared directly at the courageous young woman, now sitting at the back of the room, and said, "Leadership is about integrity, justice, and the courage to stand up for each other. I am so grateful that today I had the opportunity to witness an Upstander."

The power of standing up for each other takes great courage, but it lies at the very heart of what makes us human. Compassion and tolerance don't always come in the packaging we might expect. They are not always dressed in beautiful clothes, wearing smiles, or garbed in religious attire, nor are they always found in those who talk about good deeds. Sometimes they can be discovered in those who are unsuccessful—hobos, drug addicts, the poor—or even in cheaters, liars, and swindlers like Oskar Schindler. All of these people, in moments of truth, are capable of finding their humanity and standing up for others. Upstanders hold the true power for change and the key to survival for all of us.

Surviving the Color Gray

There are no words to describe Auschwitz. Our language is weak, and the words we know can't describe something that others cannot know. When Rena thinks of Auschwitz, she thinks of gray. The sky was gray, the air was gray, and even the ground was muddy and gray, despite the snow. The camp was near a swamp, so insects and rodents were everywhere. The skin of the prisoners was gray. There was no grass, no birds—no life. Just gray death. Gray ashes that had been people floated in the air. Hair and bones lay in piles that had not completely burned in the furnace. Rena's eyes filled with tears as she described these piles. "It is the image of the hair that gives me great pain. Our hair became clothes for soldiers, the removal of our hair humiliated us, and the hair that floated in the air was the reminder that death was coming."

Rena and the other women from Schindler's factory were in Auschwitz for three and a half weeks, which is a long time, considering that "it was a factory for killing." As soon as one transport train came, the previous round of people were killed.

One day, a day like all the others, a guard told them that they were leaving. Rena recalls thinking that it was just another cruel game. She didn't believe they would leave—nobody left Auschwitz except through the chimney. But when a female guard took them back to the showers and gave them new clothes, a glimmer of hope surfaced.

Rena stared out the window of her tidy suburban home in Florida as she thought about that day. She smiled bleakly and said, "I wonder where my shoes are now. The shoes that held the picture of my father." Then she began to rub her arm. "Those of us with the 'KL' on our arm, Schindler Jews, entered the boxcar. But this time there were places for us to sit, and the train was actually heading away from Auschwitz. It was the only train ever to leave Auschwitz with people who were alive." Rena feared that at any minute the guards would pull them all out of the boxcar and not allow them to leave. But as the engine roared and the train pulled away, she heard her father's voice: "Hold on to hope—the world will save us."

When the train arrived in Brinnlitz, it was dawn on a very cold day. The doors opened, and Rena saw the top of a green Tyrolean hat with a feather on the side. It was Oskar Schindler, standing on the platform in his shiny boots. He wore a long coat and had a cigarette in his mouth. Schindler had bribed the guards at Auschwitz for the return of his workers. The cost of their lives was a bag of diamonds. When they exited the train, Schindler looked at them and said, "The soup is waiting for you."

Rena looked at me and raised her arms. "I was saved along with 1,200 Jews because of him," she said. "He stood up. He saw us."

We All Need Upstanders in Our Lives

In a recent interview, Steven Spielberg commented that we all need Upstanders in our lives—people who are willing to take a risk, see what is hard to look at, and then take a stand to defend what is good and fight what is unjust. Not surprisingly, Rena identifies Oskar Schindler as an Upstander in her life. But she quickly added that many other people stood up for her too—people whose names she never knew: the guard who gave her the gift of a smile, a gesture telling Rena that she had been seen; the guard who allowed her to say good-bye to her father before he was killed. She also identifies her mother as an Upstander, one who kept Rena alive, physically and emotionally, during and after the war, with her kindness and cheerful disposition—despite everything that they had been through.

Rena believes that the many students she has spoken to over the past thirty-four years, students who write to her about projects they are working on to prevent bullying, are Upstanders too. "We all have the power to make a difference—it just takes courage," she said. She smiled and added that when she is asked about courage, she does not think about being fearless. "I was very afraid all the time. But when I stood up to the guard when she slapped that girl's face, I felt free." Courage gave Rena power over her fear and hope in the face of despair. "I didn't save anybody's life, but I think we all can save each other in some small way," she added. "We simply need to stand up."

All of us need to learn the power of human connection and the value of our differences. Rena's story is a cautionary tale. It tells us of the danger of seemingly subtle and innocent words, of snap judgments about those with whom we can't identify. It tells us how pernicious the blame and hate that we learn from each other can be. The "other" versus "ourselves," "them" versus "us," our distrust of differences and diversity—Rena's story shows us how dangerous these feelings are. Most of all, her story demonstrates the destructive power of silence—silence about injustice, prejudice, and hate.

Upstanders not only stand up to injustice, they also model a life of service to humanity through small gestures. One such role model is Patti Schaefer, the mother of the news anchor Stefani (Sissy) Schaefer, whom we met in Chapter 4. Patti Schaefer worked as a model in New York the 1960s. When she had her daughter, she founded a performing-arts and modeling school in the basement of her home, so that she could keep working and still be a fully-present mother. The fashion industry is notorious for showcasing anorexic models with photoshopped appearances, thus contributing to the poor body image held by many young girls. Sissy's mother, in contrast, wanted to teach women about inner beauty, confidence, and compassion for each other, by running her modeling school in a different way.

Sissy watched and listened as her mother coached young girls. "I can remember many girls who were, by modeling standards, overweight, unattractive, with ill-fitting clothes—and my mother taught them how to feel beautiful and valued," she told me. She recalls many occasions on which her mother would pack up some of her clothes or buy new clothes and then deliver them to homes in the community, telling the girls that it was part of belonging to the studio. "I am so proud to be her daughter," Sissy said. "She taught me about morals, compassion, and standing up for others. She is my Upstander."

Gratitude Gives Us the Courage to Stand Up

When Rena asked me about people who had acted as Upstanders in my life, I thought of my grandmother. At 104 years old, she still challenges me on almost a daily basis to step into gratitude. She sees gratitude as a protective shield, a kind of Teflon that allows pain, loss, and anger to glide over us without leaving lasting scars of bitterness and hate. The active process of choosing gratitude arms us with the courage to stand up for others. Though she is only 4 feet 11 inches tall, my tiny Polish grandmother—Nana—still insists in her scratchy voice that we must all respect differences in others and lead with tolerance.

Throughout my college years, I used to sit at Nana's kitchen table and listen to her stories. She was raised by poor, Catholic, Polish immigrants, who made a living as farmers. The fourth oldest of seventeen children, Nana lived through poverty and prejudice. Children in her school frequently bullied and humiliated her and her siblings for wearing tattered clothes and carrying rusty lunch buckets. They would spit on and them and call them "hayseeders"— a derogatory word for poor farmers.

"People made assumptions and judgments without really knowing us," she told me. "They blamed us for being poor because my parents had too many children or because they thought we were uneducated and stupid. They didn't bother to know that my parents had so many children because they followed the Catholic rule of no birth control, or that we could only get an eighth-grade education because to go to high school cost money. Once you get to know people and understand their life story, it is much harder to judge and be cruel."

My grandparents vowed to do their part in protecting others from the hardships that they had endured. True to that promise, with only a middle-school education, my grandparents opened a restaurant and became very successful. They held credit tabs for families who could not pay for their meals in their entirety. They bagged up leftovers after the restaurant closed and gave food secretly to people who they knew were going through hard times. And, once a week, they opened the restaurant to anybody who wanted to come and eat for free. They called it a "hot-dog party." Nana explained, "We didn't want people to feel embarrassed or ashamed of eating for free—like they were receiving charity. We wanted them to eat with dignity, so we called it a party."

Nana continues to live a life that reflects tolerance and the importance of defending others. She reminds us how easy it is to judge others when we don't know them. But once we walk in their shoes, sit at their dinner table, hear what they confess to God, and learn about their life experiences, it becomes much harder to judge. As Nana approaches her 105th birthday, she continues to push us to defend and support each other. She frequently says, "Service to each other is why we are on this earth—it is what gives us life."

No act of defending or supporting another is ever insignificant. An Upstander understands that seemingly small acts can have a lifelong impact. As a recipient of one of those "small acts," I understand the reverberating power of knowing that you are valued. Whenever I am asked about my success, my confidence, and my resilience, I tell the story of a nun who saw something worthwhile in me as a teenager and who later, as a psychologist, challenged and inspired me to go out into the world and make a difference. We met her in Chapter 8, when I shared her story to show how painful it is when people refuse to see us for who we really are but choose to use easier labels instead.

Dr. Deborah Plummer—known as Sister Phyllis Marie back when I was a teenager—stood up for me and taught me about giving voice to those who are silent. She has spent over thirty years studying diversity and inclusion. She teaches, consults, writes, and educates. But most of all, she models a life of authenticity. She is courageous in her self-examination and the correction of her biases and prejudices, and without judgment she guides others to do the same. Debbie stopped being her own bystander and stepped firmly into her black shoes—but not shoes that she thinks represent what other blacks are wearing or what her white friends will like. They are the shoes of a Jamaican and African-American ex-nun, psychologist, writer, professor, leader, wife, daughter, and friend.

Margot Stern Strom, who founded the organization Facing History and Ourselves, was the first person to write and talk about the idea of Upstanders. The term is used extensively in FHAO's textbooks and study guides. Margot sees Upstanders in history, in her students and teachers, and in the books she reads. But when asked about her personal Upstanders, she quickly identified her family—in particular her parents, Fran and Lloyd, who taught her about being a citizen and the importance of political participation. "They created a learning environment in our home that taught us to care deeply about social justice," she said. The books on Margot's shelf give her comfort and guidance as she reflects on the idea of standing up with moral courage. For Margot, being an Upstander means wanting to know what happened in our history and then finding the courage to understand why it happened—that is how we face history and ourselves.

The concept of being an Upstander is gaining traction across the country. Upstander programs are taking hold in middle schools as part of anti-bullying campaigns. College campuses are establishing Upstander programs that teach civility in debates and dialogue. Standing up against social injustice, bullying, hate, and violence takes courage, but even just one person has the power to create an immense ripple effect of social change. Being an Upstander is the antidote to indifference. Indifference kills our will, our compassion, our gratitude, and our humanity. Standing up for others and allowing others to stand up for us is the antidote. So Stand Up.

CHAPTER 10

—— ✃ ——

Conclusion: Becoming an Eyewitness

"Few are guilty, but all are responsible."

— ABRAHAM JOSHUA HESCHEL, *THE PROPHETS*

THE ROOM GREW quiet, and for the first time I noticed that it was getting dark. A faint light shone through the blinds as the sun dipped down past the horizon. I had been talking with Rena Finder for almost six hours. I reached over and clicked off the camera and tape recorder.

Rena looked exhausted. We both sat for a moment and took in the quiet of the room. I couldn't find any words to say. After each story that she told me, I had wanted to respond but felt acutely aware of the tears I was holding back. I was afraid that if I cried I might unintentionally put her in the position of needing to comfort me, and I was also fearful that once the tears started they would be hard to contain. In the silence I glanced at the photos of Rena's family, then and now, sitting on the coffee table.

As I reflected on everything I had heard, I felt emotionally drained. Rena's stories, her images, her thoughts—they were not words in a history book; they were memories of her actual experiences, and they still lived within her. I wondered how this elderly woman sitting before me could continue to tell her painful stories and revive those nightmare images—again and again and again. I started to worry that maybe our conversation had not been a good idea.

Later, as we sat next to each other on the white sofa, with her memories recorded and her photos back in the album, I reached over and took her hand. I asked her what she would do with her evening, after I left. I wondered if I should call somebody to be with her. Was there a neighbor or friend nearby who could come over? I continued to hold her hand. In the dark room she seemed so frail. I asked her, "What will happen with all the memories that we have forced back into focus? I'm worried about leaving you after all that we have stirred up."

She held tighter to my hand. "I will live with these images, the feelings, and the thoughts for a while, until they settle back to the place where they reside." She forced a smile and then let go of my hand. We continued to sit quietly. It was clear to me that the resilience of her daily life co-existed with the ever-present wounds inside her. The ten-year-old girl and the elderly woman were walking together in her big-girl shoes.

The night sky was getting darker, and it was time for me to leave. Rena insisted on walking me out to the driveway. It was an unusually cold night for Florida, and I urged her to stay inside, but she insisted on coming out with me. She made her way slowly down the stairs and through the garage to the driveway, where we waited for a driver to take me back to the hotel. As we stood there the wind picked up, and she snuggled into her sweater. Despite my renewed suggestions that she go back inside, she insisted on waiting to see me get safely into the car. Her kindness overwhelmed me.

At last the vehicle pulled into the driveway, and I started to walk toward it, turning around for one last good-bye. She stood there smiling, but her face seemed sad and her eyes heavy. I tried to fight the urge to cry, but the tears started to flow, and I could not stop. I placed my bags in the car and then went back to hug this incredible woman one last time. I thanked her for sharing her story with me.

Rena hugged me tight, then gently pulled away. Her hands remained on my arms as she looked deep into my eyes. She saw the tears. As I met her gaze, my mind flashed through all that those eyes had seen—still see. I felt such a strong connection to her, and yet it was still hard for me to understand what she had experienced.

Her grip on my arms grew a little tighter. "Thank you for listening and hearing my story," she said. "Now, whatever you choose to do with it is up to you. For me, I know it was heard. You are now an eyewitness to what happened, and my story will have life in you."

The Pain of Knowing

As the car pulled away, I felt a deep heaviness settle over me. I was exhausted. My legs felt weak, and my mind seemed numb. I felt drained of all thought. I sank into the backseat and couldn't remember a time when I had ever felt so tired. I thought about calling my husband, to let him know that I was heading back to the hotel, but I couldn't bring myself to pick up my phone. I felt emotionally paralyzed and unable to think. All I could do was watch the streetlights moving past the window as the car moved onto the highway.

My driver was a man in his mid-forties, with a stocky build, a bubbly personality, and a kind smile. He had helped me put my camera equipment in the car, and then he had waited patiently as I returned for my final good-bye with Rena. Now, settling in for our long drive, he began to make smalltalk. He talked about the unusually cold temperature and his day's travels. He glanced a few times at me in the rearview mirror as he spoke.

I didn't want to be impolite, but it was impossible for me to engage in idle conversation. I continued to stare out the window. He cheerfully kept talking, trying to engage me in discussion by asking where I was from and whether I was staying long in Florida. I heard myself say that I was from Cleveland and that my visit to Florida was just a quick trip. He nodded and told me that he was from Cambodia. He talked about his family and his reasons for coming to the United States. I heard his words as if they were a background noise. I felt only half-present in the car. As if in the far distance, I heard him ask if I was here in Florida to visit my grandmother.

With those words, an image of my grandmother flashed into my mind: Nana sitting in her chair and wishing me a safe trip to Florida, her parting words an expression of hope that I would learn something important from Rena that I could share with her when I got home. Then came an image of Rena's grandmother, teaching the little girl multiplication as she sat on the edge of the bathtub, then cleaning the dirt and debris from Rena's hair just moments before the guards led her away to her death. It seemed hard for me to breathe, as if the air had been sucked out of the car. I reached for the button on the door and slid the window down. The cold air sent a chill through me but also gave me my breath back.

After a few moments I noticed the driver looking at me in the rearview mirror. He repeated his question. I thought it would be easier just to say yes, I was there to visit my grandmother, in the hopes that it would end the conversation. Instead I heard myself telling him the real reason for my visit, my interview with Rena.

The car fell quiet. I worried that he hadn't heard my response or was no longer interested in smalltalk. At last he said softly, "She is a brave woman to talk about the horror of genocide." After that he looked straight ahead and continued to drive. The remainder of the forty-five-minute ride was silent. I thought about his words and wondered what he knew about genocide, and what they both knew about death.

Empathy: Standing in Her Shoes

When I returned home to Cleveland, late in the evening on a Saturday night, I realized that what I desperately needed was a good night's sleep to recover from the long, emotional trip. I would return to my routine and get organized, and then this dreadful feeling would pass. My thoughts darted ahead to outline a plan. I opened up my calendar and did a quick review. Tomorrow was Sunday, and I would use the day to unpack, do laundry, and listen to the audio-tapes of the interview. Then I would construct an outline to use later, when I started writing on the following weekend. My schedule for the upcoming week was filled with clinics, appointments, talks, and hospital consulting. Also scattered into the week were business and personal lunches and a plan to play golf with a friend. I was back to my usual routine, my usual life. I fell asleep.

The next morning, over coffee, my husband began to fill me in on things that had occurred while I was gone and plans for the days ahead. Household issues, plans with our girls, chitchat, funny stories about the neighbors. I felt disconnected from the conversation. I didn't care about those things; I didn't feel like laughing, I couldn't participate in the discussion. Eventually I started to cry. I felt restless in my own skin and in my own mind. Rena's words still rang in my head, and her images were vivid and clear in my mind's eye. There didn't seem to be any room for housecleaning, or our neighbor's antics, or golf, or work. None of that seemed to matter in the context of what I was remembering.

I went into my bedroom and closed the door—and I remained in there for the next four days. I canceled everything on my calendar. With pauses only to shower and to eat the food that my husband quietly brought in and set on the nightstand, I listened and re-listened to the audio-tape of Rena's words, and I began to write. But throughout those long days and nights, what continued to haunt me was my conversation with Rena in the driveway.

"You are now an eyewitness," she had said. I wanted so much to understand what that meant. An eyewitness by definition is "a person who has personally seen something happen and so can give a first-hand description of it." That didn't seem to apply to me. I hadn't actually seen anything. But she had stood in her driveway with her hands on my arms, looking squarely into my eyes, and she had not only called me an eyewitness but charged me with the responsibility of informing others. To give life to her story. I did not understand.

At first I told myself that it really wasn't an important element to the story I wanted to share about Rena, so I pushed on with my outline of the concepts and details that had filled her interview. But something wasn't working. I typed and then deleted. I drafted outlines and threw them away. I would wake up in the middle of the night, seeing an image that brought me to tears, and then I would push it away. I would sit with my laptop, staring out the bedroom window. Rena's words filled my head and created such a great sadness in me that it blocked my thoughts from forming and from making their way to the page.

Then I decided that I simply could not write this story. I put the computer away and packed up all my notes and put them in a folder. I climbed back into bed. This was not a story that I could tell. I felt ashamed of myself for opening up this elderly woman's wounds for nothing. I felt inadequate and small. I realized that this was a story for an experienced historian or a professional writer to tell. I had failed Rena and myself.

Finally, as I lay there in bed, I thought about Rena in her white dress with the red flowers. I remembered her sad eyes brightening as she described that dress and how she had felt when she put it on for the first time. I wondered if my video footage had captured that sparkle in her eye. Glancing at the video recorder on the shelf, I decided to watch the video-tape of the interview. For the last several days, I had been using my audio-tape of the interview, since it was easier to use when transcribing, and so, up until that moment, I had not watched the tape.

The Eyewitness

I put the video-tape in and hit play. There was Rena. I watched her telling her story. On the screen, I saw an elderly woman seated in a chair, holding her frail hands in her lap while her sad eyes often looked off into the distance—an elderly woman with a faint red patch on her forearm. But as I continued to watch, I saw more and more clearly a young girl with thick, beautiful hair, wearing a big smile and a pretty white cotton dress with red flowers. I heard an elderly woman's words as she described experiences filled with terror, loss, humiliation, and suffering, but I also heard a little girl describe hope and gratitude for simple kindnesses and compassion. I felt pain when I watched the little girl with the long braids struggle to comprehend why nobody saw her or heard her when she cried, screamed, and suffered. I experienced her shame when she realized that her crime was being a Jew.

I saw a little girl leave behind her pretty shoes, tucked neatly under a bed that she would never see again, and I watched her put on her warm, practical, big-girl boots and shoulder her courage. I saw her humiliation as she stood naked in front of others, as cruel things were done to her body and her mind. I screamed when the doors were slammed shut and she waited in terror for the gas to be turned on—for death to come. I cried when I watched the elderly woman sob as she shared her powerful and lingering guilt for escorting her innocent baby cousin to her death. I felt deep shame in myself for never bothering to know, to learn, or to talk about the power of hate and prejudice that lives in all of us. I heard the ticking pocketwatch in my ear and felt the warmth of Rena's father's embrace as he said good-bye to her in that cold prison cell. I stared at the images on the screen and in my mind. And then it struck me. On that cool afternoon in Florida, in the living room of an incredibly brave woman, I had become an eyewitness.

I had witnessed the heavy eyes of a woman as she looked back to a remote place in her memory, reliving the horrors of her past. I would never lose the image of her hand as she rubbed the spot on her arm where an ID tattoo had once existed, from a time when she had been reduced to a number. I had watched her frail elderly hands as she stroked photos of people she loves—people who now live only in her mind.

Now I realized that Rena, with all her courage and strength, had invited me into her world. She had challenged me to own the responsibility of being an eyewitness—to walk in her shoes and view intolerance through her eyes, to feel the raw pain of terror in her words, to taste the bitterness of indifference, and to hear the silence of hate. I am convinced that when she put her arms around me in the driveway that day, Rena knew the blessing and the burden that she was placing on me. She understood what I could not comprehend in that moment. To be an eyewitness would require the courage to stand up to my fears and be fully present—to see, hear, and know, and then to do what is right. It would take the most difficult and painful kind of courage: moral courage.

Courage Is a Moral Choice

Courage, like a wave hitting a shore, has the power to create change and overcome obstacles. And, like waves, courage can never stop. Once we unleash it and learn to embrace it, it remains a steady, rhythmic current that carries us forward. Courage is extraordinarily forceful, and when used for good it creates the same quiet, reflective, and tranquil feeling that fills us when we listen to waves hitting the shore. Courage transforms.

Several years ago, on February 27th, 2012, just before 8:00 am, I hugged my seventeen-year-old daughter Katie as she left to drive herself to school. A short time later, I was just grabbing my coffee and searching for the remote to turn off the TV when breaking news flashed across the screen. There had been a shooting at our local high school, and all the surrounding schools were on lockdown. I dropped my coffee and ran to get my cell phone, my mind racing with thoughts of Katie driving to school. I needed to get to her. She picked up the phone on the second ring, and before I could say anything she started to cry. "Mom, did you hear kids were shot in the cafeteria in Chardon? I just got a text. They're saying that one of them is dead!" The shooter had run from the building, and police were closing roads and searching the area. Warnings flashed across the television, instructing everyone in the area to lock their doors and stay inside. They had identified the shooter and were showing pictures of him on the screen, describing him as armed and dangerous.

Katie had turned around and was on her way back home when my phone rang. The local television station wanted to do a live interview with me from my home, to talk about what was happening and what people should do to keep calm and help their children cope. It was hard to focus as the horror unfolded. The day was filled with chaos and fear. Then, finally, the shooter was captured. The streets of our quiet little town were filled with fire trucks, ambulances, helicopters, and media trucks.

Reporters and camera crews pushed through the crowd as parents in terror rushed onto the scene to reach their children.

In the days that followed many questions remained unanswered, but what we did learn was that a seventeen-year-old student had entered the school cafeteria at approximately 7:30 am with a .22-caliber handgun. He fired off ten rounds of ammunition and left three boys dead and one permanently paralyzed. Our community was in shock. Prayer vigils were held, and memorials were placed around the school. Several days after the shooting, in an act of solidarity, students, flanked by parents and friends, marched arm in arm from the center of the town square back to their school. The sidewalks were lined with students and parents from nearby schools, carrying signs and flowers and wearing shirts that read "One Heart Beat."

In the days, weeks, months, and years that followed this tragic day for our community, we searched for answers that would never be found. The unthinkable, unimaginable, and unpredictable had occurred, and we were shaken to our core. Our sense of control and security was replaced by feelings of vulnerability, fear, and anger. What I realize now is that, in the midst of our shared pain, we had all become eyewitnesses. We were courageously standing in each other's shoes—and it hurt.

Those who were literal eyewitnesses to the shooting and trauma inside Chardon High School suffered exposure to horrible images that they could not erase and thoughts that recurred endlessly in their minds. They were attacked by fears that they might never see their loved ones again, mixed with guilt and the irrational belief that they could and should have done more to try to save those who died. They experienced flashbacks to the event with all of their senses, as if it were actually happening again— flashbacks triggered by a sound, a smell, or a visual reminder of the incident. When I spoke with them, it became clear that witnessing the trauma had changed them. But it wasn't just those who were in the building who were changed; it was all of us.

Our local media—camera crews, reporters, and anchors—had to investigate and tell the story of this horrific tragedy. They each had a job to do, but it was personal and painful; this was our town, our children, our friends, our shared pain. They too struggled with the images they saw and the stories they heard, and they wrestled with their own fears as they listened to and retold the stories with compassion and grief.

We as a community were forever changed by the tragedy. As a psychologist, media contributor, neighbor, mother, and friend, I watched courage in action. After a trauma, our natural desire is to fix it in some way. Sometimes we assign blame and search for a place to put our anger, or we try to distract those who are suffering by encouraging them to think about something else. But people who have witnessed trauma either directly or vicariously, through hearing, seeing, or imagining the scene, need to be given an opportunity to tell their story. They need to feel confident that those who are listening can "handle the information." They may need to describe the incident several times, including what they were thinking and feeling. As fellow witnesses, we need to dig deep, finding our courage to listen and to walk beside them as they venture down the dark path of remembering. We need to walk with them in their shoes.

Grab the Power of Opportunity

As I stared at the video of Rena, I thought about the power of one. What if Schindler had taken the easier path of closing his eyes? What if Rena had never shared her painful story with thousands of children in schools over the past thirty years? How different would history and the future be if those opportunities had been missed? What if each of the brave and amazing women who shared their stories with me for this book had chosen to remain silent? More and more, it became clear to me that each of us becomes an eyewitness when we find the courage to step into each other's stories, empathize with others' emotions, and bear the responsibility of knowing and acting on what we have heard.

We each have the opportunity to use our moral courage and become an eyewitness to the devastating consequences of indifference, judgment, loss, prejudice, and hate. As an activist, not only did Rachel Maddow see suffering and death as her peers died of AIDS, alone and in shame, she then took the hard road to make a difference and be an eyewitness and an Upstander. Through her work as an educator, author, and diversity expert, Dr. Deborah Plummer continues to bear witness to the subtle racial prejudice that exists in all of us. She bravely steps into opportunities to raise awareness and promote respect for diversity. Margot Stern Strom created an opportunity to change how millions of children study history—by adding a moral component—after battling through the difficulties of being raised as a white girl in the segregated South, where racism was not discussed or taught in the classroom, just lived. Margot, an eyewitness to both racism and anti-Semitism, decided to take the first step, seizing one small opportunity to teach a history class in a different way.

Our voices and actions can become the stones in the water that create ripples and then waves of change—and throwing the stone starts with a single opportunity. An opportunity to look and really see ourselves, both our weaknesses and our strengths. An opportunity to recognize our underlying beliefs, which sometimes lead us to devalue ourselves through words like "imposter" and "inadequate." An opportunity to risk judgment and humiliation as we bravely become our true authentic selves—fully visible to ourselves and others. Most of all, an opportunity to act as eyewitnesses to the destruction that arises from using labels that separate us from each other. We have an opportunity to be eyewitnesses to the power of making it right, even just for a moment. And because we have that opportunity, we must stand up. We must not simply observe hate but demonstrate human kindness. We must find the courage to step into and then walk in the shoes of other people and see life through their eyes.

A young high-school student from Facing History and Ourselves said it best: "We all have these elements within us, the ability to be a perpetrator, a bystander, or a hero. This class says you have a choice. It prepares you to do the right thing. By teaching us to acknowledge the suffering of others and do all we can to stop the violence that causes the suffering. That is all you can ask of yourself."

We have the ability to step into the power of human connection without losing ourselves or feeling threatened, to acknowledge our fears, and to find our resilience as we cope with and rise from tragedy. Through sharing her personal and painful story, Stefani Schaefer inspires us to live in our moments, to cherish today, to hold tight to faith, and to support each other. It takes exceptional emotional courage to step into our own big-girl shoes and cope with trauma and loss, and it takes even more courage to remain in those shoes and stand firm when pain, humiliation, and hardship hit us from the blind side. We need to embrace the opportunity to step into these moments because, when they are all stacked together, they become our life stories.

We must also stand tall, dig deep, push through fear, and step into the shoes of others. Respecting a different point of view without feeling that our own has been challenged requires strength. Hate and judgment are easy—it takes very little intellectual energy to make assumptions and to distrust others. Finding meaning and value in each other's differences is the harder way forward, but ultimately it allows us to help ourselves as well as others.

I started down the path of this book intending to investigate how successful professional women actually became successful. What opportunities and strategies had they employed along the way? Here is what I learned on my journey. If we want to be successful women, we must face our fears and insecurities by letting others see us with our talents, flaws, and inadequacies fully exposed. We need to exhibit our true, authentic selves, filled with a healthy mixture of weaknesses and strengths. Despite fame and fortune, a successful woman still stands tall in her own original shoes—not the plastic, pretentious ones that come with fame.

A successful woman realizes that strength and resilience come from allowing others to hold her up when her shoes no longer provide the support she needs. She takes the opportunity to give to others when her own pain becomes too much to bear, and if she encounters another person's suffering, she takes the opportunity to slide her feet into that person's shoes and walk, no matter how painful it is. A successful woman takes the opportunity to look honestly in the mirror and then into the eyes of another, to become an eyewitness to our shared humanity.

All the stories in this book—stories about feeling like an impostor, embracing resilience, acknowledging our invisible biases, and becoming Upstanders—lead to one lesson: we are better off, and the world is better off, when we become eyewitnesses. An eyewitness sees the broken, fragmented shadows in the eyes of those in pain, hears the silence and feels the humiliation of those who are marginalized and tortured by contempt and prejudice. She carries the burden of knowing that there is no easy fix or quick bandage to heal many wounds, but she is willing just the same to take each small opportunity to make a difference, to become an Upstander. Becoming an eyewitness is a painful journey—stepping into our humanity and into the shoes of other people forces us to confront and face many things about ourselves. But what it says to the person whose shoes we are standing in is that they have value and are not invisible.

The words of the scholar and activist Rabbi Abraham Joshua Heschel, in his book *The Prophets*, continued to ring in my head long after I had put away the video camera, the tape recorder, and the computer: "Few are guilty, but all are responsible." Through the gift of empathy, we can discover our purpose in life—our responsibility to each other. In the end, the truest measure of a successful, well-lived life is revealed when others step into our shoes and tell us that we have been seen.

Now you are an eyewitness—what will you do?

About the Author

DR. LORI STEVIC-RUST, PhD, ABPP, holds a doctoral degree in Psychology and a Master's degree in Community Counseling. She completed an internship at Henry Ford Hospital in Detroit, Michigan, with specialty training in clinical health psychology. She has been awarded a Diploma from the American Board of Professional Psychology in Board-Certified Clinical Health Psychology (ABPP).

Lori has worked in the field of clinical health psychology for twenty-five years, serving as the current Medical Director for senior services for Lake Health and an international consultant for dementia services and care. She is the President of the Board for the Lake County Council on Aging and of the advisory board for the Alzheimer Association and the Center for Dialysis Care.

Over the past twenty-five years, Lori has been a regular on-air media consultant and contributor on psychological topics, having made her debut on one of the country's longest-running morning shows, "The Morning Exchange." In addition, she hosted a cable talk show entitled "Best of Health TV." The half-hour show provided viewers with information from local experts in the medical and psychological fields on a variety of topics, including heart disease in women, Alzheimer's disease, new advances in minimally invasive surgeries, and depression.

Lori has contributed to Women's World and Fitness Magazines. In addition to this book, she is the co-author of The Stop Smoking Workbook: Your Guide to Healthy Quitting (New Harbinger Publications, 1993); Heart Therapy: Regaining Your Cardiac Health (New Harbinger Publications, 1998); Treating Depression in the Medically Ill (New Harbinger Publications,

2000), and a memoir on aging with gratitude, Greedy for Life (Integrated Health Publications, 2013), written with her 104-year-old grandmother. She is the author of the "Dr. Lori" column that appears in Cleveland Business Connects magazine and the national PS Magazine. She is also a regular blogger for The Huffington Post.

Lori is a sought-after national keynote speaker on clinical and inspirational topics in healthcare, healthy aging, and women's issues. Her infectious enthusiasm, wealth of knowledge, engaging style, and warm sense of humor have led to many organizations naming her "best speaker." She has received the Corporate Keynote Speaker of the Year award.

Lori has been recognized as a Woman of Achievement by the YWCA and received the Professional Advocacy Award from the Consortium Against the Exploitation and Abuse of Seniors. She volunteers her time mentoring women who have been victims of abuse, exploitation, and violence, helping them to discover their own strength.

Lori is a proud member of a five-generation family. She lives in Cleveland, Ohio, with her husband, Jay. They have two young adult daughters, Sarah and Katelyn. Lori is a chocolate addict and an avid Cleveland sports fan—which by definition makes her an eternal optimist.

You can learn more about Lori by visiting her website, www.doctorlori.net.

References

Brown, Brene (2010). The Gifts of Imperfection: Let Go of Who You Think You're Supposed to Be and Embrace Who You Are. Center City, MN: Hazelden.

Hough, Lory (Winter, 2015). "Facing History, Facing Herself." *Harvard Ed. Review Magazine.*

Maddow, Rachel (1994). "Identifiable Lives: AIDS and the Response to Dehumanization." Honors Program in Ethics in Society. Stanford University.

Savickas, Mark L. (1989). "Career-Style Assessment and Counseling." In *Adlerian Counseling: A Practical Approach for a New Decade*, 3rd ed, ed. T. Sweeney. Muncie, IN: Accelerated Development Press. 289-320.

Savickas, Mark L. (2005). "The Theory and Practice of Career Construction." In *Career Development and Counseling: Putting Theory and Research to Work*, eds. S. D. Brown and R. W. Lent. Hoboken, NJ: John Wiley & Sons. 42-70.

Seligman, Martin E. P. (1991). *Learned Optimism: How to Change Your Mind and Your Life.* New York, NY: Pocket Books.

Seligman, Martin E. P. (1996). The Optimistic Child: Proven Program to Safeguard Children from Depression & Build Lifelong Resilience. New York, NY: Houghton Mifflin.

Seligman, Martin E. P. (2002). Authentic Happiness: Using the New Positive Psychology to Realize Your Potential for Lasting Fulfillment. New York, NY: Free Press.

Seligman, Martin E. P. (Spring, 2004). Can Happiness be Taught *Daedalus*.

Smith, Lillian. (1978, reissued,1994). *Killers of the Dream*. New York, NY. Norton.

Stern-Strom, Margo (1994). *Facing History and Ourselves. Holocaust and Human Behavior*. Boston, Ma. Facing History and Ourselves Foundation

Made in the USA
Charleston, SC
06 December 2016